LIVE AS LONG AS
YOU DARE!

A Journey to Gain Healthy, Vibrant Years
Special Edition for RAADfest 2018

LIVE AS LONG AS YOU DARE!

LEONARD W. HEFLICH

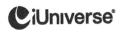

LIVE AS LONG AS YOU DARE!
A JOURNEY TO GAIN HEALTHY, VIBRANT YEARS
SPECIAL EDITION FOR RAADFEST 2018

Credits for author photo: Natalie Napoleon, Allure West Studios

iUniverse books may be ordered through booksellers or by contacting:

iUniverse
1663 Liberty Drive
Bloomington, IN 47403
www.iuniverse.com
1-800-Authors (1-800-288-4677)

ISBN: 978-1-5320-5524-9 (sc)
ISBN: 978-1-5320-5525-6 (e)

Print information available on the last page.

iUniverse rev. date: 08/03/2018

PREFACE

This book is about living. If you want to live a longer, healthier life, this book is for you. You can be any age to benefit from this book. Age is only a number, and often a state of mind, neither of which we should permit to limit our expectations. We need to dare to live longer if we are going to do it. We need to dare to live healthy, vibrant lives, regardless of our current age. Age is an artificial barrier that we must dare to break through. If you are twenty, then why not dare to live for another hundred years? In forty short years, you will be sixty. What condition do you want to be in when you get there? Nurturing and developing your healthy practices now, will enable you to arrive in great condition, ready for another fifty or more active years. And the best part, is that we don't have to wait to enjoy the benefits. The changes that we are able to make in diet and lifestyle today will produce benefits that we can enjoy now.

If you are eighty, why not dare to live for another fifty years, or longer? It will take active steps to make this happen. Most people incorrectly believe that their health is what it is and cannot be changed. We believe that some people have good genes and are healthy, while others suffer and live in a diminished state for uncontrollable reasons. The fact is that our genes account for only a small part of our health. Practices and attitude are more instrumental than we think. Attitude will play an important role in this book and in our journey. The first mistake we usually make is accepting our health as it is. The second mistake is not doing something about it.

And often, the third mistake is taking drugs to 'correct' it. We don't want to go there. We want to take active responsibility for our health, learn as much as we can about practices and technology that can help us, and adopt a healthy routine that will nurture and develop our health, so that we can live longer, healthier lives. It is not an accident or good luck. We must dare and then do it.

When I talk about taking steps to maintain your health, I am assuming that you have the capacity to be healthy. If you were healthy at some point in your life, but have lost it in some ways, there is hope that you can stop the further progression of disease and perhaps even take steps to reverse it, in order to restore your healthy state. I am not talking about diseases for which a cure doesn't currently exist, but rather about preventable diseases, such as heart disease, hypertension, diabetes, obesity and many forms of cancer. These diseases have a common set of root causes, and are avoidable, if we are aware of and make the necessary changes in our behavior and lifestyle. This is the route we want to take. I realize that we are not accustomed to thinking of these diseases as being preventable, because we are not aware of the common causes. We can change this. The prize is large, while the cost and risk are low. We will want to learn as much as we can about our particular health issues and identify the root causes. Then we will take steps to eliminate or reverse them.

> For every complex problem, there is an answer
> that is clear, simple and wrong.
> -H. L. Mencken

Much of this book is based on my own personal journey to learn how to take care of myself. As I write this, I am sixty-five years of age (notice that I didn't say old!), basically healthy, with occasional aches and pains, but have discovered during my research into this book that I was well on my way to becoming diabetic and hypertensive, like too many people today. Writing this book helped me to realize these facts about my own body, even though no one, including my own doctor, had warned me. I have read, experimented, observed, theorized and learned how to improve my own health, making significant improvements in blood glucose control and blood pressure in less than a year. I am stronger and feel better than I have in decades. I will share what I have learned, and hope that you can benefit by making similar changes and improvements in your health.

There isn't one change, there are dozens, perhaps hundreds of changes, each of which makes a tiny impact, but when combined and directed towards our vision, add up to make a powerful change. It helps when dealing with big, intractable problems, like aging, to break it up into small, bite-sized pieces that we can manage. Then as we find a solution to each little piece, we make that change part of our routine. We can commit to making one change a week, for example, so as not to overwhelm ourselves with change. You will be amazed after a year of effort how much progress you can make. Our goal is to get off of the death spiral, where we gradually gain weight, lose muscle tone, and lose control of blood glucose and blood pressure, with the result that we reduce activity, and experience further deterioration of bodily functions in a declining spiral. Wait a second – isn't that what happens during aging? Yes and no. Yes, if we stay on the death spiral. No, if we choose to reverse it by losing weight, doing more, building muscle, improving blood glucose and blood pressure control, with the result that we are able to do more and build bodily functions in an ever-improving virtuous cycle. This is where we want to be!

You have to apply yourself each day to becoming a little better.
By applying yourself to the task of becoming a
little better each day over a period of time,
you will become a lot better.
-UCLA Basketball Coach John Wooden

Before I started writing this book, I spent a lot of time educating myself about the existing published studies. There are literally thousands of journal articles and several $500 books to invest in. What amazed me is that the answers to most of my questions were already studied and published. Some were published over ten years ago. And yet, I had not seen the results of these studies reported or reviewed anywhere, and I consider myself to be a well-informed person. After all, this was my career. Even worse, friends and family members were not aware of the results of these studies or how they could help themselves by incorporating the learning into their own lives.

I am not a Doctor or even a Nutritionist. I am a problem solver. I have spent my forty plus year career as a chemist and a food scientist, studying the relationship between diet and health. It is the kind of complex, multi-factored problem that I love to solve. There are many pieces to the puzzle, which do not fit neatly together, and much of the information we have is incomplete or even wrong. Butter is bad; butter is good. Coconut oil is demonized as a poison, then is vindicated by real research and ultimately becomes a health food and cure! We're told that eggs and cholesterol are clogging our arteries, so we stop eating eggs and take drugs to reduce cholesterol, only to learn that our bodies make more cholesterol than we can ever eat and the low-fat diet we went on was the real root cause of our imbalanced blood chemistry. And on and on. Need I say more? We will discuss what we know, what we don't know and what we can theorize based on what is observable, even if we don't fully understand it. If there is a conflict between what I say and what you hear from your doctor, I suggest that you discuss it with your doctor, and if that doesn't resolve the difference, then follow your doctor's advice. Doctors are starting to learn more about the microbiome and the impact of diet and lifestyle on health. Let's look forward to the day when doctors will prescribe a high fiber diet for hypertension relief instead of a drug. The suggestions I make in this book are based on what is published in the scientific literature and on my own personal experience. Use this as a starting point for your own investigation into what will work best for you.

> The doctor of the future will no longer treat
> the human frame with drugs,
> but rather will cure and prevent disease with nutrition.
> -Thomas A. Edison

My plan for this book is to take a journey from where we find ourselves now to where we want to be. In order to get 'there' we will need to take many steps. There will be uncertainty and the need for us to ask questions, be observant and learn. We will need to consider where the 'there' is that we would like to arrive at someday. The good news is that the possibilities are expanding rapidly, and will accelerate in the near future. I suggest that it is better to think and act expansively and not confine ourselves to a diminished future, limited by drugs, restrictive diets and low expectations. I won't tell you what to eat, but focus on how to eat. I will not discuss drugs or medical procedures. I am not a fan of restrictive diets, as avoiding groups of foods can be unhealthy by depriving us of beneficial nutrients, and the evidence supporting the benefits or possible harm is weak at best and will take at least thirty years for the science to be done. The evidence will show that prognosticating based on incomplete data, is how we got into this mess in the first place. I'm not going there.

We will examine the forces that drive us, and present enough nutrition science to enable us to better manage our diets and achieve a healthy body weight. We will talk about diabetes and related diseases in order to consider what is causing these. We will collect souvenirs along our journey and these will become the hundreds of little changes that we make in our lives in order to maintain or even build our strength. Like any good journey, it will change us. It will make us aware of new possibilities and open us to new ways. Let the journey begin.

An interesting piece of trivia is that my family emigrated to the US in 1854 from Darmstadt, Germany. 'Darm' means 'intestine' in German, so Darmstadt is intestine city. Ironic perhaps that the intestine has become the focal point and root cause of my investigation into staying healthy. Like the saying that all roads lead to Rome, all of our health issues lead back to the intestines. We all live in Darmstadt!

> Our food should be our medicine and our
> medicine should be our food.
> -Hippocrates

I hope that this book is informative and compelling enough to motivate you to dare to live a longer and healthier life and give you some ideas on how to do it.

DEDICATION

I dedicate this book in honor of, and to the loving memory of, my best friend Leonard E. Burger Jr. He struggled his entire life with obesity, eventually succumbing to diabetes and heart failure. He had a very big heart, but not big enough to deal with obesity and diabetes.

I am saddened not just with the loss of my friend, but with the reasons why. Why did he die? Who or what killed him? Did he commit suicide? In a sense, we all are responsible, because we are not, or seemingly cannot change the path we are on. On the other hand, much of the advice that we have been given over the past thirty years, from well-intentioned but misinformed activists, media and experts, was wrong and often harmful to our health. This has put most of us unknowingly on the wrong path. Only recently, for example, we have learned how wrong it was to reduce fat, while unavoidably increasing sugar consumption. My friend died from bad nutritional advice. In a way, this is a murder mystery, and we are all characters and potential victims in the story. It is our choice.

I have had to accept the heavy burden that although I can help myself, I may not be able to help others, including my best friend, without their desire. His journey is over. Ours is just beginning. I sincerely hope that this book gives you some information that will allow you to help yourself to live a healthy, vibrant, extended life for as many years as you want. For as long as you dare.

ACKNOWLEDGEMENTS

Many people have helped inspire me to write this book, some by their good example, and some by not so good! By people who have spent their careers working to improve our understanding of aging and nutrition. By people who love me and support me.

Thank you especially to my mentors, coaches and supporters:

Leonard E. Burger Jr.
William H. Knightly
Dale Kuhn
Dr. Otto Siegel
Carolina Maria Brose
Vianet Galan Mendez
Marilyn Ann Heflich
Lynda, Adrienne and Brian

CHAPTER 1

LIFE EXTENSION – THE LAUNCHING PAD FOR THE JOURNEY

The concept of life extension is relatively new. Jim Strole and Bernadeane Brown started talking about it in 1968 when they cofounded the Coalition for Radical Life Extension. They have pioneered the shocking concept that death is not inevitable. We die because we either allow it or actually want it. Perhaps you have had the experience of being with a person when they were dying. The mind may give up, but the body wants to live, fighting up until the last breath. The opposite also happens, where the person gives up and mentally chooses to die, especially when they have lost a beloved spouse. We are raised in a culture where death is considered to be a part of life. That may be a healthy way to cope with death, but not a good way to extend life. If we want to extend our healthy lives, we must start by believing that it is possible, and then dare to do so. Jim and Bernadeane turn the tables on aging and death by challenging the culture of death. If death is not inevitable, and we can take active steps to extend our lives, would we take them? Given the rapid advance of technologies that already exist with many more powerful ones to come soon, maybe we should do what we can now so that when those powerful new technologies become available, we can still be alive enough to benefit. We may actually be the first generation to dare to live as long as we want. Read Jim and Bernadeane's book, *Living Without Death: The Experience of Physical Immortality*[1]. It will shock you and inspire you to start the journey to extend your healthy life.

Modern day western medicine has done a great job of extending our unhealthy lives, largely by treating the symptoms of disease after it is too late to prevent it. This may be better than dying or suffering, as people did before modern medicine, but since the drugs treat symptoms, not the root cause, we may feel better, but not get better. The side effects and interactions, are often worse than the disease itself. This is not where we want to be. We want to extend our healthy lives with cure not care. To do this, we must identify and eliminate the causes that underlie the illness, so that further treatment is not required. This is where we want to be. Healthy living for an extended period of time, without drugs or disease. We can do this if we listen and support our bodies' natural, healthy mechanisms. We have ignored or confounded these mechanisms with stress, antibiotics, lack of exercise, poor diets, lack of sleep and relaxation, lack of exposure to the sun, lack of exposure to nature, etc. – in essence bad practices and bad attitudes.

> If you are depressed, you are living in the past.
> If you are anxious, you are living in the future.
> If you are at peace, you are living in the present.
> -Lao Tzu

There's not much sense in extending our life if we are only gaining additional years of debilitating illness. The goal of extending our lives requires that we are healthy enough to enjoy an active and vibrant life. Being healthy doesn't only mean the absence of disease, but being fit and able physically, mentally, emotionally and spiritually. Achieving all those dimensions of health will keep us busy. Being healthy is table stakes in life extension. But it won't happen just by wishing or even daring. We must do it.

> In nature, there are neither rewards nor punishments--there are consequences.
>
> -Robert Green Ingersoll

The Technology of Life Extension

There has been a lot of activity in the development of life extension technologies over the past 30 years. Some of these technologies are powerful and ready to be implemented now. Others with tremendous potential are still in the experimental stages and will take another ten years or more before being ready for the market. We can learn about these technologies and avail ourselves of the ones that are ready and relevant to our personal needs. Failing to do so could be a huge opportunity missed. There is no single technology or solution that will successfully extend our healthy lives. There are many different technologies, each targeted on a different cause of aging, that together can synergistically combine to give us an extended healthy life. We will address some of these technologies later in the book. Others are beyond the scope of this book, such as: stem cells, telomerase, bioactive peptides, Growth Differentiating Factor, and hormonal balance. If you really want to keep up with the latest technologies and advances in life extension, attend the annual RAAD Festival (Revolution Against Aging and Death), organized by the Coalition for Radical Life Extension, held in San Diego each year in September.

What is Aging?

Aging is considered to be a natural and normal process of programmed senescence and loss of function that happens to living things. If we look around the animal kingdom, we find that most animals exhibit aging and death and therefore, we consider it to be 'normal'. However; there are cells in our body that do not age, meaning they show no evidence of senescence or decrease in function with time. These cells are in our reproductive system. There are animals that do not age as well. Flatworms, Planaria, bacteria, yeast and fungi do not age. They continue to divide and live without limit, or until something else eats them! Cancer cells do not age. Aging, therefore, is not universal. And perhaps not even inevitable. Our goal is to identify and understand the root causes of aging, so that we can take steps to slow them down, stop them or even reverse them.[2] Aging is a complex and intractable problem, that is made more obscure by misinformation, lack of information and a plethora of cultural traditions that prepare us for death instead of life.

We live in a culture of the past, defined around the concepts of aging and death. The way we talk, the words we use, the way we think, the way we plan, are all derived from a culture of death. We are forced to 'retire' from work, when many of us actually don't want to stop working.

We make a 'last will and testament' to plan for what happens to our assets when we die. We live our lives according to rules that were designed to control our behavior in this life so that we achieve reward in the next life. We move into fifty-five plus communities to be isolated with other 'old' people, trying to enjoy our diminished existence while waiting to die. Our bodily functions deteriorate but our doctor tells us that this is 'normal' for our age, rather than considering a proactive approach such as hormone replacement therapy, or changes in lifestyle that could stop or reverse the loss. We become diabetic, overweight, hypertensive, hypercholesteremic and our doctor prescribes drugs with life threatening or mind numbing side effects, instead of helping us make changes in our behavior that could have the same result without the negative side effects. We become 'senior citizens'. We dress like 'old' people. We get defined and define ourselves as 'old'. Aging is inevitable, the calendar relentlessly marks the passage of days and years. But getting old and dying are not the inevitable results of aging. We actually plan and choose to get old and die. It's the way it's supposed to be, so why fight it? We fight it because we can and because we want to live.

> Let us endeavor so to live so that when we come
> to die even the undertaker will be sorry.
> -Mark Twain

Ernest Becker in his masterwork *The Denial of Death*[3] points out that "the idea of death, the fear of it, haunts the human animal like nothing else; it is a mainspring of human activity – activity designed largely to avoid the fatality of death, to overcome it by denying in some way that it is the final destiny for man." He later states "There are 'healthy-minded' persons who maintain that fear of death is not a natural thing for man, that we are not born with it." Our culture and our behaviors are deeply rooted in death, based on the belief that the 'healthiest' way to deal with the reality of the death of our loved ones and eventually of ourselves, is to consider death to be a natural part of life. If we can believe that our dead friends and family members are actually not 'dead' but merely have transitioned to a different state, we can avoid some of the anxiety of missing them. We can deny death, accept it as our destiny, or live without placing artificial limits on what is possible, while neither denying nor accepting death. We choose life instead of death.

There are many factors that combine together to cause what we observe as aging, including:

- Immune system decline of function and eventual failure
- Hypertension (inability to maintain healthy blood pressure)
- Diabetes (inability to control blood glucose)
- Decline in the ability to heal
- Failure to thrive (loss of the will to live)
- Accumulation of damage from oxidative stress

- Circulatory failure (heart disease, arterial blockage, hardening of the arteries)
- Loss of muscle quantity and tone
- Dropping hormone levels and imbalance
- Dropping levels of bioactive peptides
- Slowing metabolism that results in weight gain and obesity
- Loss of mental acuity and ultimately dementia

We cannot deny that these factors are real and cause real decline in bodily function over time with eventual death. The questions we need to consider are: are these factors normal? Are they inevitable? Do we have to accept these declines in bodily function or can we do something about them? We cannot stop aging, but perhaps we can avoid getting old. There are technologies available and steps we can take now to extend our healthy lifespan.

Disease and the Metabolic Syndrome

There is an epidemic of disease that has been raging for the past thirty years globally and continues to worsen. The diseases include: diabetes, hypertension, depression, heart disease, obesity, stroke, cancer, food allergies, autoimmune diseases and PCOS (polycystic ovary syndrome).[4] The worst part is that almost all of us, regardless of age, are on the path to contract these diseases. We call it the progression of old age, as if the consequences were expected and inevitable. But even young people are on the path and already are experiencing health issues in spite of being in 'good' shape. Most of us are in denial and choose to ignore the early warnings until the disease state is reached and drugs are prescribed.

We diagnose and treat these diseases in isolation as if they were not connected, but we now know that they are connected. Gerald Reaven, in 1988 called it the Metabolic Syndrome, by proposing a common set of causes that connect these seemingly unconnected diseases. The picture that is emerging, shows that these diseases are linked to an underlying set of common causes. It is complicated and difficult to explain or even imagine, and will take decades for the complete scientific evidence to emerge.

How did we get into this mess in the first place? Basically, it all started in 1985 with a Denver millionaire named Phil Sokolof, who became the first successful food activist. Mr. Sokolof had a heart attack and asked his doctor why it happened and what he could do about it. His doctor explained that it was due to a diet high in saturated fats. Phil did some reading about it and discovered that many of his favorite processed foods were high in saturated fats, but even worse, the saturated fats were from imported tropical oils like palm and coconut. Sokolof took out full page ads in the major newspapers, accusing food companies of killing Americans to save a few pennies on the ingredient cost by using cheap, imported tropical oils, that were high in saturated fats, when they could be using domestically produced soybean oil, that was healthier, instead. The food companies immediately reacted by replacing the tropical oils with partially hydrogenated soybean oil. This was low in saturated fats, however; the partial hydrogenation process that was used to process the oil to make it functional and stable, also produced trans fatty acids. No one knew what the health impact of these would be at the time. Ironically, years later when the research was done, we discovered that the trans fats actually caused heart disease, while the saturated fats they replaced, did not. In any case, tropical oils came out of our diet and trans fats went in. At the same time, it was concluded that fat, not just saturated fat, was the cause of heart disease, so we went on a low-fat craze. Products were reformulated to remove or reduce fat, with the unfortunate result of increasing sugar. Low fat diets became popular. In hindsight, we did everything possible wrong. The production of trans fats via partial hydrogenation has since been banned and removed from our diet; and fats in general and saturated fats specifically, have been shown not to cause heart disease. The result is that butter, cocoa butter, coconut oil and palm oil are now considered healthy and are back in out diet.

The real culprit all along was sugar, and by reducing fat and increasing sugar in our diet, we made things worse and started a huge upswing in obesity and the diseases of the Metabolic Syndrome. Good intentions and overzealous extrapolation of data resulted in disease and death for millions of people. We made a lot of mistakes, and we still have a lot to learn. We now know that high amounts of sugar in the diet is part of the problem, but let's avoid the temptation to think it's that simple. We need to be careful not to demonize sugar, gluten, carrots, or any other food or group of foods, as we demonized fat and saturated fats in the past, as we could unwittingly create the next wave of disease.

Where am I to go now that I've gone too far?
-Golden Earring, 'When the Bullet Hits the Bone'

The diseases of the Metabolic Syndrome are related and stem from similar causes. We don't have to accept them and can take active steps to prevent them, allowing us to live longer, healthier lives without these diseases.

Vision

In order to support our daring goal of living longer, healthier lives, we are going to do something that we probably have never done before. In fact, it is something that very few people have done before or needed to do. Because the technology and practices supporting healthy life extension are advancing so rapidly, there are many people alive today, even those currently in their sixties and eighties, who are likely to live productive lives for another fifty years or more. We will need a vision in order to make that happen. Only Toyota has a fifty-year vision!

Yesterday I was clever, so I wanted to change the world.
Today I am wise, so I am changing myself.
-Rumi (13th century Persian poet)

To help us define our vision, let's start with a question that is radical and new. Would we live our life differently today, if we knew that we had fifty or one hundred more healthy, active years to live? Most people currently in their sixties and eighties, consider that they have at best a ten or twenty-year horizon ahead, with the last ten likely spent going to doctors, taking lots of pills and not feeling like doing very much. This is not the horizon that I am talking about. I'm talking about energetic and active years, where we are healthy and vibrant enough to do what we want to do and enjoy it. Leave the walker and cane at home – we will not need them!

> If I knew I was going to live this long, I'd
> have taken better care of myself!
> -Mickey Mantle

What will we look like when we arrive at our visionary goal? Will we be diminished in health and vibrancy or will we maintain our activity level? Is it actually possible for us to be better and stronger than we are today? If our health doesn't limit our physical and mental activities, what kind of goals will we set?

> "Would you tell me please, which way I ought to go from here?"
> "That depends a good deal on where you
> want to get to" said the Cat.
> "I don't much care where" said Alice.
> "Then it doesn't matter which way you go" said the Cat.
> "So long as I get somewhere" Alice added as an explanation.
> "Oh, you're sure to do that", said the Cat,
> "if only you walk long enough."
> -From Lewis Carroll's Alice's Adventures in Wonderland

Our vision doesn't need to be very detailed, and it doesn't need to describe a destination or even a specific goal. We may surprise ourselves and get to the destination sooner than we planned or even worse, when we get there we may not know what to do next. Maybe when we get there we won't be ready to die! Life is best considered to be a journey and not a destination. Our vision should describe the journey we want to take. Envisioning a journey that is robust enough to guide us for the next fifty or one hundred years is truly a new adventure. We are among the first to attempt to do this. Therefore; we will be pioneers cutting a new path and developing new tools. The good news is that since no one knows how to do this, we can have some fun and make it up as we go. Let's get together in fifty and one hundred years to compare notes. Pretty heady and exciting stuff!

A personal vision can guide us towards a desired, healthy future state. Why vision small? We want to dare to aim high. We want to live our lives with intensity and intentionality. The intentionality comes from our vision. The intensity comes from our commitment to the vision. We want to create a BHAG – a Big Hairy Audacious Goal as described beautifully in *Built to Last: Successful Habits of Visionary Companies* written by <u>Jim Collins</u> and <u>Jerry I. Porras</u>[5]. Making the vision big, audacious and a little scary (that's the hairy part!), makes it interesting, challenging and worth our extra effort to achieve. Visioning small is a waste of time and effort. Visioning big will inspire us and those around us to dare to do big things.

> "The size of your dreams must always exceed
> your capacity to achieve them.
> If your dreams do not scare you, they are not big enough."
> -Ellen Johnson Sirleaf

A vision is the most powerful way to direct long-term behavior, like a compass that always points north. We know what direction we want to head in, even if occasionally derailed from our path by the stuff that life throws at us. We have no way of knowing what challenges will confront us in the future, but with a vision, we will not lose our way. We will always know which way to go and what choices to make, enabling us to make the little and big decisions along the way. A good choice is one that is aligned with and helps us get closer to our vision. Other choices that are not aligned with our vision will slow us down, dilute our efforts and drain our vital energy.

> Where there is no vision, the people perish.
> -Tao Te Ching

A vision also helps us stay focused on the future, not the past. The past was great and it is gone. The only time that anything ever happens is now. We want to drive our 'now' based on where we want to be tomorrow and in the future. If every step we take brings us closer to our vision, and we keep at it for some time, we will eventually get there.

> Yesterday is gone.
> Tomorrow has not yet come.
> We only have today.
> Let us begin.
> -Agnes Gonxha Bojax (Mother Theresa)

Without a vision, we are not only lost, but we are listless too. We don't know where to go and we don't know what to do. This is a recipe for disaster. We will lose interest in life and lose our love of life. Once this happens it is a short distance to giving up. It's time to consider what we want to do (present) versus what we have to do (past), and what we will need to do in order to be successful (future). Limits are a thing of our past. We want to live in the moment, every single one of them for the next fifty or one hundred years, as Eckert Tolle describes in his seminal book *The Power of Now*[6]. And we want to make each moment count and be valuable. Fifty years sounds like a long time, but to put it into perspective, it is only 18,250 days. That is a small finite number!

> The search for happiness is one of the chief sources of unhappiness.
> -Eric Hoffer

Purpose and Play

Consider two seemingly mutually exclusive concepts: purpose and play. We need a purpose to our lives in order to motivate us and excite us. And that is where the play comes in. Play is fun and fun is good. Play brings in the excitement. We want to devote our lives to some purpose that is meaningful to us, and also have some fun while doing it. Play is the grease on our gears and bearings. Without play we get grumpy and tired and eventually fail. Like a motor running without oil, it gets harder and harder all the time to do what we used to do easily. There just seems to be more friction, more obstacles in our way every day. That hill we used to climb has gotten a lot bigger lately. We have less and less tolerance for distractions and difficulties. This is not where we want to be. We want to live our lives with intensity and intentionality. Intentionality is having a purpose and a reason to live. Intensity is the energy we put into living so that we get the satisfying and meaningful experiences we seek.

Dr. Stuart Brown has written a serious and playful book on exactly that subject: *"Play: How It Shapes the Brain, Opens the Imagination, and Invigorates the Soul"*[7]. In the book, he shows the importance of play in the development of young animals, including humans. Actually, especially in humans, because we have a more extended adolescent period than any other animal. Play is the method used by all animals to develop their brains and social skills. But play is important for other activities as well, including social interaction, bonding, mating, friendship, building trust and work. Play is so important, that animals are willing to risk their lives in order to play. Dr. Brown describes how baby mountain goats play by jumping from rock to rock, but occasionally they slip and fall to their death. Their playing allows them to learn how to jump to safety when a predator is chasing them, a very useful skill. There is a cost to this learning and they are willing to pay it. Play is not just for kids (Ha!). Adults need to play too. In fact, Dr. Brown shows that adults need play almost as much as adolescents, for different reasons. Adult play is less focused on developing social skills than in creating and maintaining social ties. A relationship without sufficient play becomes stale and stiff. The interactions become rote and joyless. A little teasing and friendly banter between people reduces tension and creates social bonds. People who play every day are happier. They find the joy in life. They create and share their joy for life with those they interact with. These are great people to have around and we want them as friends. Play keeps them and us young. If we want to extend our healthy lives, we must play every day.

Play puts joy into our work and our purpose. This is not drudgery; it is fun and exciting. We want to achieve our vision because it is meaningful, but more than that, we want to work on achieving our vision because it is fun and we make it fun. The key is making it fun. Making it fun doesn't happen by accident. We must do so on purpose! See how purpose and play fit together nicely?

A great way to give work a purpose is by doing work that contributes to some greater good. Helping others can be very satisfying. Applying a special skill or experience that we have to solve a problem, teach, write or create can be rewarding, especially if appreciated. Most schools and universities gladly accept knowledgeable people as guest lecturers or aides. I find that there is no shortage of work when you are not looking to get paid! My pay comes from their appreciation for my experience. Of course, this is a benefit that I enjoy after having worked for many decades. Young people are very smart and open to learning, but may lack the real world experience to put what they learn in school into a useful context. This is where an experienced person can contribute.

Some people have hobbies to keep them busy. There is nothing wrong with this, unless there is no goal or vision to give the work a purpose. Without a vision to drive the hobby, there is no purpose, except to keep busy. We may be able to motivate ourselves for a while, but eventually we will lose interest and the work will become drudgery. Work that has meaning can get us out of bed in the morning. It can sustain us when there are difficulties. Challenges become hills to climb instead of mountains that block our way. Many people have a strong need to create. Hobbies can be an effective outlet to express our creativity and satisfy this need. A nice painting or photograph is a great gift, or looks great hanging on the wall, giving us satisfaction every time we walk past. I hang up everything on the walls of my office and elsewhere! The joy I get from seeing those theatre tickets from a play we saw, is better than leaving them sit overlooked in a drawer. Going to that play was a pleasant experience that I want to remember often. You will probably agree that creating and remembering good experiences is more satisfying than buying a new gadget. The novelty of the gadget often wears out before the batteries, but the joy from a good experience lasts forever.

A vision and a purpose make what could be 'work' into 'satisfying fun'. People who enjoy what they do and have fun doing it, will never really work another day in their lives! Good work keeps us mentally and physically active, not just busy. The older I get, the more I realize the value of good work, motivated by a vision. I like to say that the most optimistic thing we can say every day is 'We have work to do'. When the day comes that we have no work to do, that will be a bad day indeed. It is similar to eating, and we will talk a great deal about diet in the coming chapters. I do not live to eat, but rather eat to live. Similarly, I don't live to work, but rather work to live. Attitude!

A vision without a task is but a dream.
A task without a vision is drudgery.
A vision with a task is the hope of the world.
-Anonymous, Circa 1730

What is Possible?

When considering our vision, we will need to consider what is possible and what is impossible, and then push the limits. First, let's consider the factors that drive our definition of the impossible:

- Where do our limits and constraints come from?
- Are we inhibited by feelings or fears?

- Do we have physical, mental or emotional limitations?
- Are we worried about failing or ridicule?
- What scares us the most about failing?
- What concerns us most about how other people think of us?

Now, let's flip it and consider the factors that drive our definition of the possible:

- Have we really thought about what is possible in our life?
- What motivates us and drives us to excel?
- What is there that we cannot do today, but if we could, it would change everything?
- What is the worst that can happen?
- How is that working for you?
- What is the best that can happen?

If the worst that can happen is failure, and we can handle it, then the worst is not so bad. Elon Musk, founder of Tesla, Solar City and Space-X is not afraid to aim very big and fail. He knows that even if one or more of his projects failed, he would still survive. But he is not planning for failure. He is planning and hiring the best people to assure success. For people like this, failure is not an option. They will have a plan B and C, ready just in case plan A flounders. With just a little luck and common sense, we won't be eaten by a lion or end up in prison! We can do better than that.

> The greater danger for most of us,
> is not that we aim too high and fail,
> But that we aim too low and succeed.
> -Michelangelo

Never listen to an 'expert' who says that something is impossible! An expert is limited by their vast but still finite experience. Their experience blinds them to the possibilities and opportunities. Francis

Fukuyama famously predicted the 'end of history' in his 1989 essay, proclaiming that the cold war was over and liberal democracy had been established as the model for the future. There have actually been volumes more history written since then, in spite of his prediction and lots more to come. What expert could have predicted in 1947 when Bell Lab scientists Bardeen, Brattain and Shockley invented the transistor, that it would replace vacuum tubes and eventually reduce the size of the device from several inches to less than five nanometers that is standard in 2017 and continuing to shrink as this is written. It was not possible to see that far ahead and therefore, an expert at the time would likely have said that it was impossible to make a device as small as is routinely done today. An expert can only stand on the hill that he or she is on. Standing on top of the hill gives them a better view than anyone else, but all that they can see is the next hill. When the next hill is climbed, it is possible to see further, but again, only to the subsequent hill. By successively climbing hill after hill, eventually we arrive where we are today. It took persistence, commitment and guts to continue climbing technological hill after hill to get to where we are today. But there is no other way. This is the power of vision. To see beyond many hills to a distant, unseen but desirable future state. The vision gives us the faith to keep on climbing hills. Taking the challenge one manageable step at a time, but always in the direction of our vision, so we don't get lost.

> The reasonable man adapts himself to the world;
> the unreasonable one persists in trying
> to adapt the world to himself.
> Therefore; all progress depends on the unreasonable man.
> -George Bernard Shaw

The world today is bursting with opportunity. The rate of change in almost every industry is faster than ever and still increasing. Where there is change, there is opportunity. When the ground is stable, it is impossible to move large objects like buildings. But when the earth is moving, as in an earthquake, even large buildings and mountains move. Today the foundations of our society exist in a perpetual earthquake. The ground they are built on is now soft and moveable. Changes that would have been impossible to consider a few decades ago, today are happening and can be made to happen, by people with vision and purpose.

The journey of one thousand miles, begins with a single step.
-Lao Tzu

Attitude

I already told you that attitude was going to play a big role in this book. Having a positive attitude about life and our current situation is going to be critical to our future success. If we have a positive attitude, we can weather the difficulties and occasional failures. We can endure some hardships, especially if those events are the result of efforts towards achieving our vision. A positive attitude can also mean that we take a bad situation and change it for the better. We don't just put up with failure or pain, we actually do something about them. In order to be happy and successful we need optimism and pessimism in the proper balance. Without optimism, we become bitter. Without pessimism, we become fools.[8]

The pessimist sees the difficulty in every opportunity;
the optimist, the opportunity in every difficulty.
-Winston Churchill

Attitude can impact our behavior and health, both negatively and positively. Some people in clinical research studies get well, believing that they are getting a breakthrough medicine, even though they are in the control group getting sugar pills. This is the placebo effect. The opposite effect is called the nocebo effect. People feel worse or get ill, believing that a drug or treatment will harm them, even though the treatment is harmless or they haven't received the treatment.[9] If we believe that we will get sick when we fly on an airplane, because we read it somewhere, we are more likely to get sick. People can make themselves feel better or worse, depending on their expectations and attitude.[10] If we want to extend our healthy lifespans, we will need a positive attitude. We want to take advantage of the placebo effect and avoid the nocebo.

> Don't die before you're dead
> -title of book by Russian poet, Yevgeny Yevtushenko,
> about the attempted overthrow of Mikhail Gorbachev

Why do people choose to die before they are dead? This is the power of attitude. My friend Tom Pickard told me a powerful story about his father, who was suffering from heart disease. He was a big, strong, physically active man, but heart disease was wearing him down. This was before modern medicine found ways to address the symptoms of heart disease. One day, he told Tom that he realized that he couldn't win this fight. He gave up mentally and within a few weeks he died of a heart attack. Giving up may not literally mean giving up. I have friends who have retired and when I ask them what are they planning to do in retirement, they answer proudly 'Nothing'! Or they end up spending too much time watching TV. This is not healthy and is just another way of giving up. If we want to extend our healthy lives, we need a purpose driven by a vision. We need something to do and a reason to do it. Don't die before you're dead, unless you want to.

> Ability is what you are capable of doing.
> Motivation determines what you do.
> Attitude determines how well you do it.
> -Lou Holtz

One more thing that we will need to consider all through the rest of this book is the concept of life force. Our life force is what drives us to live every day. If we are really serious about extending our healthy lives for twenty, fifty, one hundred, or more years, we will need to have a strong life force. The first step is to be aware of our life force and how it depends on our attitude. Then we must learn how to nurture our attitude and life force in order to develop and make them even stronger.

Let him that would move the world, first move himself.

-Socrates

What We Don't Want!

Paradoxically, it's easier to identify what we don't want in the future than what we want. Therefore, in the exercise that follows, we will identify some of the places and situations where we don't want to be on our vision date. We will then turn these around to help us figure out what we need to do in order to achieve the vision we do want. It's easier to envision from the negative perspective, but always better to act from the positive. Why is that? Our culture is based on avoidance. Eight of the Ten Commandments are written as 'Thou Shalt Nots'. Only keeping the Sabbath and honoring your parents are written as a 'Thou Shalt'. We probably got the same message from our parents. Even laws and regulations are written predominantly from the perspective of what is illegal as opposed to what is desired. The Declaration of Independence, by the way, is a strikingly wonderful exception to this rule!

Of course, some behaviors carry such a heavy penalty that avoidance is the only practical way to manage them. Smoking cigarettes, addictive drugs and murder are best avoided at all cost. Staying out of jail and not being broke might be worth avoiding as well. We need to educate ourselves and take the appropriate steps to avoid what we don't want while working to get what we do want.

Ignorance is no defense when it comes to regulations and laws, so we will need to be aware of these. Money is nice but it is not everything and should not be a goal in itself. I advise people that their vision should never be to make money. Making money is a result of achieving our vision, not our vision. Usually, if we are good at something and practice constructive behaviors such as sharing, collaborating, aspiring, growing, thinking, partnering, etc., the money will come as a natural consequence of our success. On the other hand, if we focus on making money at the expense of these other activities, we will either fail or be miserably rich. Not where we want to be.

Based on our culture and upbringing, which are largely based on the avoidance of sin as opposed to the commission of virtue, it's no wonder that we find it easier to envision avoidance behaviors. We will use this cultural bias to help us identify what we don't want in our vision and then flip them around to identify the positive things we want, as it is more effective to motivate behavior in a positive fashion. A vision based on avoidance does a good job of describing what not to do, but not a very good job of describing what to do. We want to focus on what to do. Lastly, striving for the good things we want to do, leaves space for some of the bad things we will want to do! Strict avoidance behavior leaves no room for a little bad to leaven the good. After all, we are not angels and really don't want to be.

I've learned from years of work in consumer research, that most people cannot identify what they want, but they have no problem describing what they don't want! We can easily come up with the usual silly answer – I want to be rich, good looking, healthy, married to a person half my age, in a beach house, without a care in the world, with no demands, etc., etc. That does sound pretty good, but it's not realistic and I don't know about you, but I would need something to do. I need a challenge and a purpose. Perfection is not happiness, it is death. Let's try a different approach.

> That which can be foreseen can be prevented.
> -Charles Mayo

Let's identify some places we don't want to be on our vision date in the future. For example: we don't want to be dead, in jail, in the hospital, in a nursing home, broke, alone, etc. It's easier to envision where we don't want to be than where we want to be. Once we have identified and eliminated the places where we don't want to be, then what is left should be places where we would like to be. Maybe not a specific place but a bunch of acceptable places. That could be a good way to start. Let's make a big list of places and situations we don't want to be in on our vision date, and then we are going to turn those around to define the places we want to be. The rest of this book will then be devoted to figuring out how we can get into those places. We will need to work at it and even change some things in our lives. But the point is, with some directed effort led by our vision, we **can** make changes and take the steps that will **enable** us to get where we want to be! Not only can we do this, but if we want to extend our healthy lives, we must do this.

Here is a list of some places we don't want to be on our vision date in the future:

- Dead
- In jail
- Broke
- In the hospital or in a nursing home
- Alone
- Cancerous
- Obese
- Suffering from inflammation
- Diabetic
- Stroke or heart disease
- Hypertensive
- Addicted
- Miserable
- Demented
- Depressed

- Unable to do the things we enjoy
- Suicidal, or at least willing to die

That's a good list to start with. Perhaps your list would be different. Let's turn each of these around in order to define **what we will do** to achieve **what we do want**.

- Living a healthy, vibrant life (that covers a lot of them!)
- Free and able to do what we want
- Active and physically capable of doing what we want
- Healthy blood pressure (not hypertensive)
- Healthy blood glucose (not diabetic)
- Positive attitude

The list of what we want is shorter, because each one encompasses many of the 'don't wants'. Notice that good looking, rich and famous are not on my list! Maybe they will be on yours. Let's get started. We have work to do!

Action

Life is what we make of it. The universe is full of energy, change and possibility. But the universe is silent. It is nonjudgmental and unforgiving. It does not take sides, nor condemn action. It is supportive, giving us all we need to develop and grow, if we choose to do so. It is a giver of life and energy. But if anything is going to happen, we must make it happen. And before we can make it happen, we must decide to do it. Assess the situation, identify the opportunities, how we can contribute, changes we can make, what is possible, what is seemingly impossible, then decide, commit and go.

Part of extending our healthy lives is to enjoy the healthy life we have. These are mutually generating feelings. If we are healthy and vibrant, we are more capable of enjoying life. If we enjoy our life, we are more likely to be healthy and vibrant and take the steps needed to stay there. It is a virtuous cycle. We want to be here!

> Unless people believe that they can produce desired effects and
> forestall undesired ones by their actions,
> they have little incentive to act.
> -Albert Bandura (Psychologist)

There are so many ways to enjoy our lives and to share that enjoyment with others. Sharing our joy doesn't diminish but rather enhances it. Purposeful work, contributing, collaborating, volunteering and teaching are great ways to enjoy life and share it. And there are others too like eating great food, traveling, or just plain relaxing. We can create great experiences for ourselves and our loved ones by traveling or by having parties. We have had an annual BBQ party at our house for the past 40 years. It has become a tradition that we all look forward to and is one of the best things we ever did. So many of our friends say – "We need to do this too". But then – you know – the kitchen needs to be painted, or the rug in the den needs to be replaced first. The result is they never have the party! I know that we will have the party in July, so if the kitchen needs painting, I had better do it in January. Or if it doesn't happen, no one will notice that it needs painting except me – so let's have the party!

> To find the meaning of life, ask 'what gives meaning to my life?'
> -Me

We need other people. We need to be part of a community in order to be healthy and extend our healthy life. Teaching and mentoring others is a great way to give back. Exposure to young people can keep us young too. We are all part of the matrix of life and need to stay connected to other people. I have always had several mentors. These were people who I respected and trusted enough to share personal problems with. They were able to help me see a different perspective on my problems. They gave me confidence that I was on the right track or guidance when I wasn't. These are the people who support us in times of need. We need mentors and to be mentors to others. We want to continue to learn and grow. Creativity is a special gift that all of us get in some measure. The need to create is strong in many of us. Part of enjoying life is allowing our creative juices to flow as they will. We all have talents, but we cannot expect to sit down at an easel and paint a picture without study or practice. We need to take some steps to enable our talent to develop and mature. Many people discover and develop their latent talent when they are older and wiser. Grandma Moses is a famous example, not starting to paint until she was seventy-eight years old. Tony Bennett has also become an accomplished painter after a remarkable career as a singer. There are lots of ways to express our creativity. One that I particularly like is finding new ways to enhance my health, strength and life force. Writing this book has been a result of that search and I hope you find it worthwhile and creative!

Life is a gift. Think about it. Why are we alive? Is there a reason or a purpose for our life? Can a universe with over two trillion galaxies be an accident? Can we be an accident? We can attempt to answer these questions or avoid them, like most of us do, because we cannot answer them or because we might not like the answer. But these questions are there. Enjoy them and actively learn how to enjoy our lives.

Hope

Human beings live on hope. Without hope we are lost and empty. Hope gives us the push we need to get over the occasional rough spot in life. It keeps our attitude positive in spite of challenges or crises that befall us. We cannot control everything in our lives, so bad things will happen to us no matter how we prepare and plan. That is not pessimism, it is reality. Bad things sometimes happen to good people, but we cannot allow those bad things to derail us from our vision and goals. We need hope to bridge the gap and bring us to a new level beyond the crisis du jour.

He who has a why to live for can bear almost any how.

-Nietzsche

Hope keeps us emotionally whole and allows us to function even when it looks futile. We stay the course towards our vision and goals, confident that the crisis will pass eventually and we will get to fight another day. But hope is not enough. We still must persist and work towards our vision and goals. Continue to nurture and develop your health even when you don't feel like it. Stay the course in spite of a temporary illness or a pulled muscle. You may need to adjust or find some new practices to help you get over this challenge. This is one way in which we grow. We pull a muscle or aggravate a joint doing what we thought was a good activity. We need to assess what happened, why it happened, what we can do now to repair it, and what we can do differently in the future so that it doesn't happen again. Maybe we should wear a supportive brace on our knee in the future when we do strenuous work involving the knee. Maybe we need to do more strength-building exercises with our knees to protect them from injury in the future. Hope tells me that there is a solution, if only I can find it. Hope tells me to persist and not accept a diminished level of activity or vibrancy. Once we stop doing something, because 'we cannot do it anymore', it is lost. This is how we get old. We stop hoping and accept a diminished physical, mental or spiritual state, which then defines us going forward. We don't want to go there!

Summary of Life Extension

As Yogi Berra once said, "The future ain't what it used to be." Our future doesn't have to be the future that previous generations had to accept, or even the one that we thought we had to accept. We have a unique opportunity to create a different kind of future, not just longer, but healthier and more active. Technology is part of it, but attitude and desire are also necessary elements. The pieces of a huge puzzle are falling into place, allowing us to envision a different kind of future. A future that is worth daring and creating.

CHAPTER 2

LIFE FORCE

Our life force is our will to live. Life is not an accident; it is highly intentional. Look around and wherever we look, there is evidence of the power of the life force. I love to garden and I collect seeds wherever I go. I have acorns from Oak trees in many different places. I've noticed something interesting when I plant them. Most of them will germinate and start to grow. Some sprout vigorously and take off for the sky like rockets. Others are more tentative, and grow slowly. And some, sprout and then stop, as if they changed their mind. I realize that seeds are highly variable and this is what drives natural selection. The vigorous seeds grow and pass on their genes to future generations. The tentative ones fail and wither away. We are no different. Some people are born with a powerful life force. These people are the doers. They are vibrant and seemingly up all the time. They attack life with vigor and good humor and are usually the most successful among us. If we want to extend our lives, we will need to take some lessons from these people in order to nurture and build our life force.

Our life force emanates from every cell in our body. It is not localized in any particular organ or part of our body. The collective force from all our cells combines to create our life force. Some people call the life force an aura or energy field. These are describing the same thing. We want to be aware of our life force and then take

27

steps to actively nurture and develop it. There are programs designed to help visualize it. Bob Monroe Associates has some excellent meditation programs to do this[11]. Our life force doesn't exist only inside of us, there are several other significant forces around us that contribute to it as well.

> I know, your Honor, that every atom of life in
> all this universe is bound up together.
> I know that a pebble cannot be thrown into the ocean without
> disturbing every drop of water in the sea. I know that every life
> is inextricably mixed and woven with every other life. I know
> that every influence, conscious and unconscious, acts and reacts
> on every living organism, and that no one can fix the blame.
> – Clarence Darrow

The following graphic identifies some of the elements of our life force and our connection to the earth, moon and sun. There is also a force emitted by the surrounding universe, but I couldn't fit the more than two trillion galaxies we now know to exist on the page. We will have to imagine those!

THE TREE OF LIFE

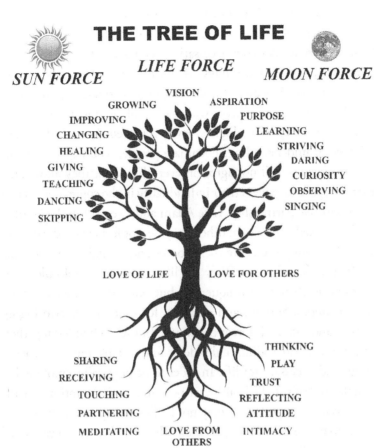

LIFE FORCE

SUN FORCE   *MOON FORCE*

VISION
GROWING   ASPIRATION
IMPROVING   PURPOSE
CHANGING   LEARNING
HEALING   STRIVING
GIVING   DARING
TEACHING   CURIOSITY
          OBSERVING
DANCING   SINGING
SKIPPING

LOVE OF LIFE   LOVE FOR OTHERS

          THINKING
SHARING   PLAY
RECEIVING   TRUST
TOUCHING   REFLECTING
PARTNERING   ATTITUDE
MEDITATING   LOVE FROM   INTIMACY
          OTHERS

EARTH FORCE   Images used with permission
          Getty iStock Images

Let's start at the bottom and work our way up the tree. The Tree of Life has roots, and around the roots are the grounding activities that we need in order to nurture our life force. Like the roots of a tree that gather life-giving moisture and minerals from the soil, and anchor it to the earth, we gather energy and stability from the Earth Force via our roots. To be fully alive and experience life in a meaningful way, we need strong roots to nurture and support us. There are many roots, starting with the love we receive and share with others. We take in spiritual nutrients from others by partnering, sharing and touch. The ultimate form of this kind of sharing is intimacy, which occurs on physical, mental and spiritual levels. Physical intimacy does not necessarily mean sex, but certainly sexual intimacy involves intense physical sharing, partnering and touch. Mental intimacy is achieved when we can share our deep, innermost thoughts with another person, without fear of judgment or criticism. Spiritual intimacy is the highest level, achieved through deep love and mutual understanding. Fortunate people, who experience this level of intimacy will not agree on everything, but they allow each other the space to express their individuality in the context of a stable and supportive partnership. Like Adam and Eve, still in the Garden of Eden, naked before each other, they do not feel exposed, trusting each other enough to share their bodies and thoughts without fear of criticism or judgment. They are like atoms in a molecule, each contributing their own uniqueness, but bonded together to create a new material. Sodium and chlorine, for example are two highly reactive, and totally different chemicals. But when bonded together, these atoms create sodium chloride or salt, a stable molecule that is benign and necessary for life. In order to be physically, emotionally, mentally and spiritually healthy, we need to experience intimacy with at least one other person. It may not be fair to expect one person to be able to give us everything we need. Therefore, we need a variety of people in our lives, each contributing a piece of the intimacy that we crave. The sum of these relationships is love. We cannot live without love in our lives – love of life, love of ourselves, love of others and love from others. If we are not experiencing enough of these grounding activities, then our life force is diminished, and we may be unstable. A strong gust of wind, in the form of a severe challenge, could knock us down. Or when there is a drought, we could wither and weaken.

Someday, after mastering the winds, waves, tides and gravity,
we shall harness the energy of love, and for the second time
in the history of the world, man will have discovered fire.
-Pierre Teilhard De Chardin

In order to have positive relationships, we need to build trust with other people. We need to have contact with people whom we trust enough to share, partner and develop intimacy. These acts are risky and we must expose our inner self to other people in order to develop intimacy. If we are closed up and unable to trust others, we cannot develop intimacy. Conversely, we need people who trust us, so that they feel free to open up to us. These grounding activities enhance our life force by giving us energy. We get physical energy from interacting with people whom we love and trust. We mutually stimulate each other to do things and be active. I often don't much feel like taking a hike by myself, although I have done it. It's far more fun to plan and take a hike with other people. We challenge them and they challenge us. We get emotional energy from others. We talk and question and tease a little. This healthy banter raises our energy level and our mood. If I'm in a bad mood, for whatever reason, I call or text my friend and she knows exactly what I need to hear to get me going again. We get mental energy from others in the form of ideas or questions. These ideas expand our horizons and help us to change and improve. There is so much going on today all around us, it is impossible and undesirable for us to try to keep up with it all. I tap into the experience of my friends, who have different interests than I do, which enables them to discover new ideas that I would never find. New ideas keep us mentally fresh and challenged. Finally, we get spiritual energy from others. When we are together, we can share our life force up close with a touch, a handshake or best of all, a hug. Hugs are a great way to share our energy with each other. We both gain and neither lose.

Love all, trust a few, do wrong to none.
-William Shakespeare

Did you know that we can build our life force by doing simple activities that create joy in our lives? When was the last time you skipped? Skipping is unlike walking or running. It is an expression of the joy of life. Skipping can enliven us and lift our mood, enhancing our life force. Simple acts like this can nurture and develop our life force. And imagine if someone sees us skipping! They may think that we are crazy, but they cannot help but share in the joy and life force we are expressing!

Only that day dawns to which we are awake.

-Henry David Thoreau

The roots of the Tree of Life are grounded in the earth and derive sustenance and energy from the earth. We can enhance our life force by tapping into the earth force. We are part of the earth. The earth is alive. It is not some chunk of dead rock floating in space. Some people call this Gaia, recognizing that the earth itself is a living organism. We are one small part of the life force on earth. All around us there are life forms, many we have never even discovered and certainly are unaware of. We dig a well one mile deep and find bacteria there. The earth is literally alive. All of these life forms emit life energy. Even inside of us and all over our bodies there are over ten trillion bacterial cells without which we could not survive. We are only beginning to understand the nature of our microbiome and its impact on our health. There is tremendous energy in all of these life forms and in the living earth. We are part of the earth and our bodies absorb energy from the earth. We can enhance this effect by being aware of it and practicing Chi Gong, where we feel the energy from the earth entering our body through our feet, progressing through each organ and body part, until it reaches the top of our head and then cycles back again to our feet, building and building. This is a powerful exercise to do every morning and if we do it right, we will energize our body and strengthen our life force.

We can enhance our attitude via meditation, thinking and reflection. Reflection on our successes and mistakes can be fun and help us to improve, as long as we don't dwell in the past. These activities focus our mental energies inward, so that we can understand ourselves. We need to pay attention to our body and our mind in order to assess our condition and discover what we need. Then we need to take active steps to care for ourselves in order to keep well and improve. Stress is one of the most destructive forces in our lives. The world, and our personal world, are changing constantly and not always in ways that we like. Other people, even those that we love, impose their will on us and cause us distress. We can feel the stress of change in our mind and in our bodies. Some of us are able to absorb the stress and not worry or seem to care. This could be positive, or they might be hiding the impact, even from themselves, allowing the stress to build inside. Others, fret and allow the stress to wash over them like a wave, knocking them off their feet. The best approach is to be aware of the stress, consider our options to deal with it in a positive manner, and then move on, not burying it, but defining and keeping it outside. Meditation and reflection are positive ways to deal with stress, while maintaining a positive attitude. We need to be like a duck – the wave might wash over us, but we maintain our balance and it doesn't make us wet.

You may want to add some other grounding activities that are important to you. I was going to add shopping! Hobbies, travel, partying, exercising, running, hiking, bowling, fishing, golf and many other activities can be part of our earth force. Recognize which ones are most important to you personally, and take active steps to enjoy and develop these.

In the leaves of the Tree of Life, I have placed the expressive activities that define us as people and allow us to enjoy life. With these activities, we enhance our life force and make life worth living by constantly growing, improving, changing and healing, just like a tree. Without these activities, we will die. These come from our vision, which drives us to aspire, dare and strive based on our purpose. We are curious, listen and learn by observing. We sing, dance, and skip with the joy of life, because it is in us and we express it in everything we do. Finally, we give to others by sharing.

On the trunk of the Tree of Life, I have placed 'Love for Others' and 'Love of Life'. These are the forces that convert our grounding behaviors into life energy. If we do not love ourselves, other people and life itself, our life force will be weak and we will die. Loving life means loving what we do and caring about it. It means loving ourselves enough to do what is necessary to take care of ourselves even when sometimes those behaviors are difficult. Loving life means loving the people we interact with, always searching for new people to bring into our lives and sometimes eliminating those who are not interested in living. The power and vitality of their life forces will combine with ours to enhance or detract. Love of Life means loving everything about life, wanting to be alive and actively living in a vibrant, positive manner.

The moon emanates a force too, that is especially powerful for women. The menstrual cycle is only one easily observable and powerful impact of the moon force on our bodies. The moon impacts the weather, the seasons and of course the tides of the ocean. All life on earth is in tune with the rhythm and energy of the moon. The full moon is known to cause behavioral changes in humans. Call centers staff up on full moons, knowing that the influx of calls will increase. The moon has a special pull on water, and thus the tidal effect. We are also composed ninety percent of water and this water feels the force and ebbing attraction of the moon.

The sun emanates tremendous energy that we can easily see and feel. Sunlight contains infrared radiation in addition to UV and visible light. The infrared is particularly healing for our bodies because it penetrates several inches below the skin to reach and energize internal organs. We should try to get ten to fifteen minutes of direct sunlight onto as much of our body as we can manage every day. The idea that sunlight causes cancer, or that we need to wear sunblock whenever we are in the sun, is incorrect. Sunburn, which is damage caused by excessive exposure to UV radiation, causes cancer. A few minutes of direct exposure to the sun without sunblock will not cause cancer and has beneficial healing properties. It also produces Vitamin D.

The earth and the moon are so intimately connected, that the rotation of the moon exactly coincides with its orbit around the earth. The moon rotates on its axis once every twenty four hours, exactly as the earth. This is why we always see the same side of the moon. By the way – the same is true for the earth and the sun. The orbit of the earth around the sun exactly coincides with the rotation of the earth. This is why at noon the sun is at its highest point in the sky every day of the year. If this were not true, then at noon on December 21st the sun would be high in the sky, and on June 21st at noon our time, it would be middle of the night. The sun, earth and moon are intimately connected. There is value in appreciating that we are part of this highly interconnected system.

Finally, there is Universe energy. The most powerful telescope built by man, Hubble, has seen two trillion galaxies, each with several hundred million stars. We don't know how many galaxies are actually in the universe, but if we can count two trillion, the real number is far larger, perhaps ten or one hundred trillion. That is unimaginable in scope. If the earth, moon and sun emit so much energy, can you even imagine how much energy comes from ten trillion galaxies? It is interesting to compare the universe outside of us with the universe inside of us. There are about one hundred trillion cells in our body, the universe inside of us. There are perhaps one hundred trillion galaxies in the universe outside of us. We have as much complexity inside of our body as exists in the universe outside. That is a remarkable concept. And you have difficulty loving yourself?

Beloved, I pray that you may prosper in all things and be in health,
just as your soul prospers.
-2 John 1:2

These forces from the earth, moon, sun and universe seem remote and even mythical. We have a difficult time feeling them directly. Our awareness of them is low and needs to be developed.

Let me tell you about a real impact these forces have on our body. Dr. Thomas Cowan has written an outstanding book on the heart and circulation system, *Human Heart, Cosmic Heart*[12]. The ancient Greeks thought that there was a special force in our bodies that made blood flow. In 1628 an English physician named William Harvey published a treatise on the circulatory system where he showed that the heart was the motive force behind blood flow in the body, not some inherent force in the body. He used science to dispel the ancient theory and this has been the conventional wisdom ever since. However; Dr. Cowan, following the work of Rudolf Steiner, showed that it is impossible for the heart to pump blood through some three thousand miles of veins, arteries and capillaries in the human body. Clearly, the heart does pump blood, but the pumping force generated by the heart is insufficient to the task. There must be some other force that works with the heart to enable blood to flow as it does. He studied trees and found that the tiny tubules in a tree carry sap from the roots to the top of a tree several hundred feet up. And trees do not have a heart or any other pumping organ. The sap just flows. Capillary action is part of the force, but is not sufficient. Cowan proposes that the force that pumps sap in a tree and blood in our capillaries is the same force. It is due to an electrical charge that is created inside the capillary by the capillary wall. Water in the blood that is next to the capillary wall is charged and has a different structure than ordinary water. He calls it structured water, because it is more highly structured, it is viscous and has the curious ability to force normal, unstructured water, of which blood is composed, to flow. The electrical charge in the structured water is responsible for the flow of blood in capillaries. This pumps blood back to the heart to enable the heart to do its job. Without the capillary capability, there is no blood flow. Where does the electrical charge that drives the capillary pumping action, come from? It comes from external sources of electrical energy – the earth's magnetic field and sunlight are the two most important. Therefore, it is electrical energy from the earth and the sun that provides the motive force to pump blood through our bodies. Our bodies also generate electrical energy, so we can survive for some time without exposure to the sun or earth energy, but at some point, we need to 'recharge'. We generate electrical charge by metabolizing glucose, which comes from a plant that produced it via photosynthesis, which is sun energy. No matter how we look at it, we are running on sun and earth energy.

You might wonder, where does God fit into this model? That is a personal decision. We all define God differently, if we believe in the existence of one at all. It seems to me that if our belief in God helps fill in some of the gaps in our belief system, then that is good and healthy. It's interesting to note how we behave when we are confronted with a crisis in our lives. Do we get depressed or despair of the situation? Do we come together with friends and family for support and get it? Do we internalize the issue and act as if nothing happened only to suffer from it for years? Do we cry or get angry? Do we pray and put our faith in God? A crisis in our lives can be a severe challenge to our life force and can derail us from progress towards our vision. If faith in God helps us, that is good and powerful healing. On the other hand, if our belief in God is excessively restricting our freedom to live our life due to avoidance rules, then it could be a liability. And don't forget the guilt driven by religion. Carrying around the guilt for our sins for the rest of our lives can be crippling. The Catholic Church got this one right – confess, take absolution, accept forgiveness and move on, without guilt.

> The child whispered, "God, speak to me."
> And a meadow lark sang.
> The child did not hear.

> So, the child yelled, "God, speak to me."
> And the thunder rolled across the sky
> But the child did not listen.

The child looked around and said,
"God let me see you" and a star shone brightly.
But the child did not notice.

And, the child shouted,
"God show me a miracle."
And a life was born, but the child did not know.

So, the child cried out in despair,
"Touch me God, and let me know you are here."
Whereupon, God reached down and touched the child.
But the child brushed the butterfly away
and walked away unknowingly.

Used with kind permission from the author,
-Ravindra Kumar Karnani

Where do you think we come from? From the earth is the simple, obvious answer. Where does the earth come from? The higher-level elements such as oxygen, nitrogen, sulfur, iron, zinc, magnesium, calcium, iodine, carbon, and sodium required tremendous energy to form from elemental hydrogen. The only place where there is sufficient energy to produce these elements is in a star. Life is not possible without these elements and they all came from a star that existed billions of years before the earth. The star produced these elements, died and exploded, spreading these elements out into space. Eventually, the matter ejected by this dying star, cooled and coalesced due to gravity into our solar system and earth. We are made of these elements. The water on earth was not here when hot matter collected and formed our planet. The earth was too hot at that point to retain water. Billions of years later, after the earth cooled and an atmosphere capable of retaining it had formed, water from asteroid impacts started to collect on the surface. All the water on earth comes from asteroids – snowballs from space. Where did that water come from? From the stars. We are ninety percent water. Therefore; we are ninety percent made from asteroids from space, and the rest from stars. It is no exaggeration to say that we are made from the stars![13]

Our life force is anti-entropy. Entropy is death. Entropy is the natural an unavoidable direction of the universe away from order, towards increasing disorder. Entropy is thought to be the clock of the universe, always pointing in the same direction, and never reversing. Heat flows from a warm substance to a cold one, never the other way around.[14] An ordered state tends to move to a more disordered state over time (my desk is a good example!). Human activity can reverse entropy for a while, but eventually it catches up. We can build a wall, but eventually it will fall down. Life is the force that builds walls and opposes entropy. A cell takes disordered molecules and puts them together to produce a highly ordered and functional cell wall. An organism combines many different kinds of cells, each with a specific function, into a highly ordered and functional structure such as the human body. The fact that these highly ordered collections of cells produce a life force and a living animal is still miraculous to us because we don't understand it, but thousands of different kinds of animals perform this miracle every day.

Women are the source of the life force among humans. Women are more in touch with the earth and moon than men. They are the only ones who can create life and give a newborn child a life force of its own. They draw on energy from the universe, sun, moon and the earth. Most religions have at least one female deity or member to connect with the female life force. Even the male-centric Catholic Church reveres the Blessed Virgin Mary and many prominent female saints, such as Joan of Arc and Mother Theresa. Men can also tap into these external sources, but most of a man's life force comes from the women in his life – his mother, his wife and friends. Men seek the company of vibrant women, with strong life forces for this reason.

We are a twig on the tree of life. We are derived from the earth, sun and stars. We cannot exist without the life-giving energy from the earth and sun. We are a tiny speck existing on a tiny speck in a tiny section of the universe, and yet, we are a part of it just as sure as it is a part of us. It is a worthy goal to be aware of these energy forces and how to tap into them to enhance our own life force. If we want to extend our healthy lives, we will need all the life force we can get!

I love the Vince Lombardi quote:
"Winning isn't everything, but losing is nothing!"
And paraphrase it for our purposes as:
Living longer isn't everything, but dying is nothing!

Be Nice to Yourself!

If we are going to successfully extend our healthy lives, we will need to be nice to ourselves! I hope that you love yourself. We will have a difficult time loving others, or loving life if we don't love ourselves. We are all we have. We are not perfect, but we can improve, if we want to. We are going to need every part of our body working together in order to live a healthy, extended life. Therefore, we need to appreciate all of our parts and all of our characteristics, including the imperfections. In fact, especially our imperfections, as these define us as a person just as much as our strengths. We need to cherish who we are and be grateful for what we are. Loving ourselves in balance with our love of others and of life isn't narcissistic. Dr. Otto Siegel[15] calls this "Extreme Self Care", because if it's going to help, we need to get good at it and take our self-care to a new, extreme level. This is about changing our lifestyle in order to change our lives. It is extreme, in that will take a lot of effort and persistence to care for ourselves in ways that we have never done before. No one knows us better than we do. No one can feel what we feel, or interpret what we are feeling to find the sometimes-hidden meaning. Doctors try to help us but often apply the same treatment to different people experiencing a common set of symptoms. Perhaps this is adequate, but it is not extreme. We need to get involved, observe, ask questions, read, experiment and learn how to take care of ourselves. Push the limits. Don't accept the standard. Go to the extremes to find a better way. Extending our healthy, vibrant lives will happen by intent, not by good genes or good fortune.

There are so many ways to be good to ourselves, to increase our joy and love of life. Being good to ourselves makes life worth extending. We will have to work hard to successfully extend our healthy lives, and to achieve our vision and goals. Why do all that if there is no reward? Life itself is a reward. Health is a reward. Doing activities that we enjoy with people we love is the icing on the cake.

A hot tub, sauna or a warm shower is a great way to relax not only our muscles but also mentally. I have a routine of stretches and yoga exercises that I do twice a day in the hot tub and shower. The warmth loosens up stiff muscles, making the stretches more effective and less likely to cause damage. Put some Epsom salt in the water to make it even better. There is a lot of evidence that frequent use of a hot tub or sauna prevents hypertension and improves circulation. It's also great for sore muscles after a workout or after overdoing the yardwork.[16]

Go get a massage! Do it on a schedule with the same person and you and they can learn what and where to focus. Myofascial therapy and chiropractic are two other ways to push and shove muscles and bones back where they are supposed to be to alleviate pressure on nerves and joints. They are very different therapies and useful for different issues. I hurt my knees by hyperextending them and spent two years in pain. Just before accepting that the next step was an MRI and probable surgery, a friend suggested that I try myofascial therapy instead. There is a myofascial therapist a mile from my house, so I went. Caran Kalish pushed and shoved my knee and the tissues surrounding it for six sessions and the pain disappeared. I work my knees hard with yard work every day. I can work with pain and did, but it's so much nicer when they don't hurt! I am now a believer in myofascial therapy and suggest that you add it to your toolkit. Keeping ourselves well and in good condition is a project that we need to take seriously and get good at.

Making time to exercise is one of the best ways to be nice to ourselves. See the section in Chapter 7 on Exercise.

Having a hobby is a wonderful way to be nice to ourselves, doing something that we love to do. The activity, if aligned with our vision, can be motivating, rewarding, and an outlet for our need to create. And when we accomplish something, it brings great satisfaction, especially if we can share it with another person.

We will need to balance the good work we must do to extend our healthy lives and accomplish our vision and goals, with time to relax and enjoy it. Find ways to relax that are enjoyable to you and the people you spend time with. Reading is one of my favorite ways to relax and I like to read on a range of subjects. Listening to music is also very relaxing. Taking a walk, especially barefoot in the grass is great. Have a party with friends, even if it's just two or three people. Make it special and laugh a lot!

Eating and drinking well is a good way to be nice to ourselves. Of course, we have to be careful not to eat too much, but we can eat well in quality and variety without exceeding our limits on quantity. And once a week, we can allow ourselves to go beyond the limits, as long as we make up for it in the next few days.

All things in moderation, especially moderation.
-Ralph Waldo Emerson

Incorporating essential oils into our daily routine is a luxurious way to be nice to ourselves. We can aspirate lavender into the air. It smells great, it relaxes us and supports our parasympathetic nervous system. It helps us sleep better and deeper. Coriander oil makes a luxurious foot massage and eliminates fungal infections. It's great fun experimenting with different combinations of oils like rosemary, clary sage, honeysuckle, patchouli, geranium, tea tree, lemon grass, thyme, eucalyptus, and many more. There are lots of great books on the subject.[17]

Another way to be nice to yourself is to always have something to look forward to. Plan a trip or a party a few months away. When it's done, plan another. Having something to look forward to focuses us on the future, which is where we want to be focused. We don't want to dwell or live in the past. The past was great and it's done. Let's look forward to an even greater future.

Whenever I do a task, I think of a way of rewarding myself, if I've been a good boy and gotten it done! The reward can be small like a cup of coffee or a beer, but it focuses my efforts and helps me persist to get it done so that I can enjoy the reward. *Zen and the Art of Motorcycle Maintenance: An Inquiry into Values* by Robert M. Pirsig[18] is a fascinating book about the human condition, and a little about motorcycles. He talks about the importance of getting up the gumption to do a task before setting out to do it and what happens when the ten-minute job that we expected, turns out to be two hours. Simple rewards can give us the gumption we need to get the job done in spite of setbacks and extra difficulties we didn't anticipate.

If we are going to live longer, healthier lives, we will need the gumption to do so. Gumption is an attitude that comes from our vision. We need to visualize our future and then develop a plan and actions around the vision in order to make it a reality. Henry Ford said "Whether you think you can, or you can't – you're right." If we want to live for another fifty years or longer, the first step is to think that we can. If we think that we cannot, then we are already defeated. Thinking that we can will enable us to find the steps we need to take to make it happen, and then actually do it. Try visualizing your longer, healthier life and see how it changes your attitude. Creating that vision and using it to guide our actions is a powerful way to make it a reality.

> For it is in giving that we receive.
> -St. Francis of Assisi

Lastly, one of the best ways to be nice to ourselves is by being nice to others. Maybe that sounds a bit selfish, and if you like we can have a side discussion on whether any human activity can be purely altruistic! However, it really feels nice to give to others, especially when they appreciate it. It is a win-win. Teaching, sharing our hobbies, even simply showing interest in another person are ways to give.

> We make a living by what we get,
> we make a life by what we give.
> -Sir Winston Churchill

Existence and Exploration

Daring to live longer will put us on a journey of exploration and discovery that starts with ourselves. We have so much to learn about ourselves. We send probes into space to take pictures and gather samples from distant planets, but we know so little about the bacteria that colonize our intestines. Do we really know ourselves? What do we see when we look in the mirror? Actually, even that is wrong, as it is a reversed image of us. This is why many of us don't like photographs of ourselves, as they are a true image of us, and not a match for what we think is us – what we see in the mirror. Are we comfortable with ourselves? We are who we are and cannot change dramatically. The first step in self-discovery is to accept what we find there.

The next step in exploration and discovery regards others. Do we really know the people with whom we live and interact? Are we interested enough in them to ask them probing questions? What do they like? What are their goals? What is their vision? These are questions that we usually don't ask. We get stuck in small talk about the weather, sports and politics and never get around to asking them how they feel about life. We don't really know the people around us.

If we are going to successfully extend our healthy lives, we need other people whom we know deeply. We need to know their vision and goals and they need to know ours. Sharing our visions is a powerful way to create positive, enduring partnerships, where we support each other to success.

Finally, we need to explore the universe around us. We are a solitary person, on a tiny planet, in a small solar system, that is part of an unremarkable galaxy, in a huge universe of over two trillion galaxies. And we think we are special? Well, actually, we are special. Among all of those galaxies, it's only reasonable to conclude that there must be other planets like earth that could support life. Life is such a powerful force; it is hard to imagine that earth is unique and alone among over two trillion galaxies. However; when we do find life on another planet, it is likely to be different from us. We may not be able to physically or even optically explore the vastness of the universe, but we can imagine the extent and power it generates. We are a part of the universe. We can explore ways to bring the energy that it emits into our bodies to enhance our life force and health.

In many ways, we are explorers on a mission to discover how we can extend our healthy lives. The word 'discover' is appropriate, as much of what we need already exists inside of our bodies or in the world around us, and our mission is to find these techniques, materials, activities and forces. We are among the first in history to take on this quest, so we should be prepared to make mistakes and for inevitable surprises. This is exciting and can be a purpose in itself. This is where we want to be!

Learning and Self-Development

If we are going to live another vibrant fifty or one hundred years, we will need to continue to learn and grow. The world is changing at an accelerating pace. We can choose to keep up or fall behind. Falling behind is one reason why people choose to die. They can no longer relate to the world around them. Often, their friends and family members have passed on, leaving them alone. They don't recognize the world anymore. They cannot understand how to use new devices and technology. They become more and more isolated and cut off from society. We don't want to go there. We want to keep up with the world as it changes. This means keeping up with technology as it develops, keeping up with our communities as they inevitably change and grow, and keeping current with the bigger world around us in terms of politics and programs. It means keeping up with our friends and having a network of people we can talk to and socialize with. We do not want to become isolated or alone in any sense.

We have to learn how to learn. Learning is a skill just like any other. If we practice it, we can get better at it. There are so many opportunities to learn today and many are available for free. Coursera is an online service that offers university level courses on almost any topic to anyone. The cost is minimal or free if you choose. The key to learning is to ask questions, to be curious. When we stop being curious, it means that we know everything we want to know or just don't care. This is death. Learning is challenge. Learning is growth. Learning is life. We choose life.

> I know of no more encouraging fact than
> the unquestionable ability
> of man to elevate his life by conscious endeavor.
> -Henry Thoreau

We can focus our learning on improving what we already know a lot about. This could be one of our hobbies, special talents or work skills. For example: maybe we are good at woodworking. We can find some books or courses on woodworking that will take us beyond what we already know. We can buy a new tool that we've always wanted or teach a course on woodworking. The best way to learn is to teach! The other option is to learn something new. Learn a language, how to paint, play piano, etc. There are lots of wonderful skills we can develop that will bring joy to us and the people we know. A friend of mine has a German heritage, and in his eighties he decided to learn how to play accordion to accompany him when he sings at the annual family Octoberfest. Al is the hit of the party.

> The illiterate of the future will not be those who
> cannot read, but those who cannot learn.
> -Alvin Toffler

Volunteering

Volunteering is an interesting and effective way to collaborate with other people and to share our experience and joy with others. The concept of volunteerism largely originated with one very influential person – Benjamin Franklin. Ben wrote a beautiful little autobiography that I highly recommend to you[9]. An interesting bit of trivia is that he wrote the original in French while he was in France cajoling Louis to support the American Revolution. In the book, he chronicles his lifelong efforts on self-improvement. He was a printer, a writer, a political activist, a humorist, a statesman, an ambassador, a signer of the Declaration of Independence, a scientist, an inventor and a community organizer. In addition, he pioneered the creation of free public libraries, volunteer fire departments, local community hospitals, local universities, and more. Volunteerism has become a unique and important part of American culture. We often don't wait for government to solve a problem; we organize and find a way to get the job done. This is very Ben Franklin! We can build upon this pillar of our society by using our leadership skills and experience to organize a group to tackle some problem in the community. It is a great way to contribute and give back. It is a great way to share our expertise and love for our community. If we want to extend our healthy lives, we need a powerful life force that enables us and makes us want to live intensely and intentionally. Volunteering can help us to do that.

Developing Our Life Force

We know so little about life. We are ignorant about the existence of life elsewhere in the universe and yet cannot imagine that in the vastness we are the only planet to manifest life. We are only slightly more informed about life on our own planet. We are just starting to appreciate the life that exists on and inside of our own bodies. We observe that life is everywhere on our planet and body. We wonder how life started. What was the spark that took simple elements and pushed them to defy the inevitable, grinding advance of entropy to increase order? This force is the life force, and it is incredibly powerful. We have this force inside of us and all around us. We can build our awareness of this force, develop it, nurture it and ultimately use it to improve our lives and health.

CHAPTER 3

NUTRITION BASICS

Extending our healthy lives will require that we understand some basic facts about nutrition and the impact that diet has on our health. Human nutrition is a complex and developing science. Food and diet depend on many factors including the availability of food, economics, seasonality, personal preference, culture, religion, social interaction, and much more. Studies on the impact of diet, therefore have a lot of variation to contend with. We talk about the Mediterranean Diet and attribute the apparent health benefits enjoyed by its practitioners to olive oil and red wine. These are likely part of the story, but stress, smaller portions, socializing, activity level and other factors are not to be overlooked.

Performing controlled studies on human nutrition is notoriously difficult as people are uncontrollable and often don't pay much attention to what they eat. In addition, the impact of diet on health often takes several decades to become measureable. The best nutrition studies, such as NHANES and The China Study involve over five thousand people and monitor their diet and health over many years. There are some problems with these studies as well to be aware of. The data collected is usually analyzed via statistical correlation, a technique that finds trends and associations in the data. Unfortunately, correlation does not indicate causality, so a positive result must be further studied to determine the true root cause of the apparent association. A famous example was the finding that coffee consumption correlated positively with heart disease. The initial conclusion was that people who drank more than three cups of coffee a day were at greater risk of developing heart disease. We now know that coffee, due to its high antioxidant content, is actually protective against heart disease and other health issues. It took twenty years for the research to be done that finally vindicated coffee, and now coffee is considered to be healthy. The mistake was caused by the presence of other underlying root causes that were not included in the study. It was eventually discovered that people who drank more than three cups of coffee per day, had different lifestyles than the non-coffee drinkers, and those behaviors were the true cause of heart disease, not the coffee.

Let's start with some basics on nutrition to set the stage for discussions about diet and disease.

Calorie-containing nutrients:

There are only three kinds of calorie-containing nutrients – carbs, protein and fat. The unavoidable consequence of this, is if we want to reduce fat intake, then we have to increase the amount of protein and carbohydrates in our diet. There is nothing else to replace the fat we remove! This is why low fat or no fat diets don't work long term. The balance of the three types of nutrients is critical to digestion and good nutrition. We cannot be healthy without these three basic nutrients, in proper balance.

Proteins:

Proteins are polymers of amino acids. There are twenty one amino acids in the proteins that constitute the human body. Eight of these are essential, meaning that our bodies are not capable of producing them. Our bodies also have no way to store protein, so eating a high protein meal today does us little good tomorrow. Any protein we ingest, that is in excess of what our bodies need today, will be converted into urea and excreted in our urine. Eating protein is a daily requirement. If we do not eat the right amounts of the right amino acids, we will not have the amino acids that we need and the body will scavenge the amino acids needed for repair by breaking down muscle, resulting in muscle loss. In a sense, using muscle as a source of necessary amino acids is a sort of 'storage' mechanism, but not one that we want to utilize. Therefore, we should pay attention to the amount and the kind of amino acids that are in the protein we eat.

Some proteins are naturally balanced according to what our bodies need. Egg protein, for example, contains the most perfect balance of amino acids of any protein source. Milk, meats, fish and soy are also very good. Other protein sources such as rice, beans, wheat and corn contain a less perfect balance of amino acids. The balance of amino acids is expressed as a number called the Protein Efficiency Ratio (PER). Egg protein, with a perfect balance of amino acids for human nutrition, has a PER of 1.0. Wheat has a PER of 0.86, meaning that it is 86% efficient. We need to consume 1/0.86 or 1.16 grams of wheat protein to get the same benefit as 1 gram of egg protein. We can and should eat different kinds of foods with different protein efficiency ratios, so that the deficiency in one food is compensated for by the excess in another. A classic example is eating beans and rice together. Rice is low in lysine, a required amino acid, while beans are high enough in lysine to compensate for the shortage, when the two are consumed together. It's not that one protein source is good and another bad, but rather that some are more efficient than others and combining different kinds can compensate for the imbalance. In the case of rice and beans, the result is that the body gets the amino acids it needs in proper balance from a diet that contains both protein sources.

Basically, protein is the building block of muscle, and there is a minimum level of protein intake required to repair and build muscle. Too little protein can result in the body breaking down muscle to liberate the required protein. We don't want this to happen. Too much protein in the diet results in high uric acid content in the urine. This could be a benign consequence, unless we also have poor circulation in the extremities of the body like toes and fingers, in which case the uric acid could form tiny, sharp crystals in the tissues, causing gout, which is very painful. The Dietary Reference Intake (DRI) for protein is 0.36 grams of protein per pound of body weight or 54 grams for a 150-pound adult. Bodybuilders increase their protein intake up to 1 gram per pound of body weight in order to build muscle, or 225 grams for our 150-pound adult. Higher levels of protein are also useful in helping us reduce fat intake and therefore reducing body fat. As you can see, recommendations range from 54 grams up to 225 grams per day for a 150-pound adult. That is a wide range. Increasing protein in the diet allows us to decrease fat and carb intake to moderate levels, which is a good direction to go, especially when we are trying to lose weight, reduce body fat, reduce stored intracellular fat, and reduce fat stored in the liver, with the goal of increasing insulin sensitivity. I suggest that we take a middle target of twenty percent of protein in a 2,500-calorie daily diet, which is 125 grams of protein. This is a reasonable target.

Fats:

Fats are used to build the walls of our cells. We cannot produce all of the kinds of fat that we need, consequently, we would die if we stopped consuming fat. Our brains are high in omega-3 fats, and since we are not able to produce certain required omega-3 fats, a shortage will have a serious impact on our health. Some of the less severe consequences of eating too little fat include dry skin and hair falling out. The optimal level of fat consumption is a balance of how much fat we need to eat in order to get the essential fatty acids with the amount of calories that the fat contains. Fats contain 9 calories per gram, which is more than double the caloric content of protein and carbs at 4 calories per gram. Protein and carbs are almost never eaten dry. Most protein and carb-containing foods have over a fifty percent water content, which increases the weight of the food and decreases the caloric content, whereas fat absorbs no water and is often eaten as is, such as in butter or olive oil. Therefore, in order to control caloric intake, we want to be careful with how much fat we eat. A moderate and reasonable goal when trying to reduce or avoid excess stored body fat, is for fats and oils to comprise about twenty percent of our caloric intake, which is 55 grams per day of a 2,500-calorie diet.

Carbohydrates:

Last and not least, carbohydrates are composed of sugar molecules linked together in different ways and in different patterns. Sugar, starch, cellulose and dietary fibers are carbs. Some carbs can be broken down into sugar while others cannot, passing into the intestines largely intact. There are many different kinds of sugars. The most common sugars are glucose and fructose. Glucose is found in corn syrup and in sucrose. Fructose is found in fruits and in sucrose. Sucrose is a disaccharide, composed of two sugar molecules linked together, one glucose and one fructose molecule, making it half glucose and half fructose. Sucrose is found in cane and beet sugar and is what we know as 'table sugar'.

Glucose is the fuel that our bodies burn, and carbs are the only energy source we can metabolize directly to produce glucose. Protein and fats must be converted into glucose in order to provide energy. The basal requirement for a human is approximately 2500 total calories per day. A bit of trivia is that this is equivalent to approximately 75 watts of electricity – so we burn about as much energy as a 75-watt incandescent lightbulb! (or 5 – 15 watt LED bulbs).

Fructose cannot be metabolized directly by the cells in the body and must first be converted into glucose. This happens in the liver, where there are enzymes to make this happen. Oddly, there is no good mechanism in the body to control the conversion of fructose into glucose, versus storage as glycogen or fat, as there is for glucose. The result is that a substantial percentage of the fructose we consume is converted into glycogen and fat, specifically very low density lipoproteins (VLDL).[19] [20]You probably have heard of LDL and HDL, which are fatty components in our blood. HDL is protective and LDL is destructive to arteries and veins. VLDL is even more damaging than LDL. This is how diets high in fructose are thought to contribute to heart disease. Fructose is in sucrose, high fructose corn syrup (HFCS) and fruit sugar. HFCS is 55% fructose and 45% glucose, similar to sucrose. The sugar in apples, oranges, bananas, berries, etc. is almost pure fructose. Apples, oranges or a banana contain 20-25 grams of sugar per fruit, mostly as fructose. The body can handle this amount of fructose safely. It is only when daily consumption of fructose goes higher than about 75 grams that there are issues with VLDLs. Don't forget that fructose is coming into your diet from several sources, including fruit, sucrose and high fructose corn syrup. Plain corn syrup is pure glucose and not an issue. It is the best and most healthy sugar to consume.

Starch is a polymer of glucose molecules. The process to break down starch into glucose begins in our mouths. Saliva contains amylase enzymes that immediately begin breaking down starch into glucose. In fact, if you keep a starchy food in your mouth, you will notice that it becomes sweeter with time. This is due to the breakdown of starch occurring in your mouth. Interestingly, trees are also made of glucose, but the glucose molecules in cellulose are linked together differently than in starch. Our intestines do not contain the enzyme necessary to digest cellulose and therefore we cannot eat trees. Termites live on wood but actually the bacteria in their guts digest the cellulose! Read a wonderful account of sugar production in plants in *Lab Girl* by Hope Jahren[21]. Think about it – trees are actually giant candy canes!

Recommendations on energy intake from carbs vary from forty to seventy percent of total calories. This translates into 800 to 1400 calories a day from carbs. Since carbs produce about four calories per gram of dry material, this is 200 to 350 grams of carbs. This sounds like a lot, but remember that all plant-based foods contain carbs. The quantity of carbs consumed should be in balance with activity level. We will talk in more detail about diet, but the basic idea is to keep fat and protein intake relatively constant, while carb intake varies with activity level. If you live a sedentary lifestyle, then you want to keep carbohydrate intake near the basal level of 300-350 grams per day. If you are a Marathon runner, then you need to eat more carbohydrates, or you will literally starve to death. The American Council on Exercise estimates that a 180-pound man will burn 17 calories per minute while running, so during a 3-hour marathon, a runner will burn 3060 calories or 765 grams of carbohydrates! This is more than ten times the normal daily basal requirement for a sedentary person of about 1.4 calories per minute. Getting this amount of energy from protein or fat will put tremendous strain on the liver and could cause ketosis, a dangerous imbalance of blood pH. Please see the section on exercise in Chapter 7 for more details.

> Everything you see, I owe to spaghetti.
> -Sophia Loren

When we ingest more carb calories than we need, the excess is converted into glycogen and fat, to be stored in anticipation of a time when we will need the extra calories. If that day never comes, meaning we eat multiple times a day, always taking in as many or more calories than we need, the fat just accumulates. We need to give our bodies an opportunity to remove some of the stored fat or we will become diabetic, overweight and eventually obese. Excess storage of fat in the liver and muscles blocks insulin receptor sites, one of the causes of insulin resistance and diabetes. Chronic over-nutrition is one of the critical causes of diabetes and the Metabolic Syndrome[22].

Fear less, hope more, eat less, chew more, whine
less, breathe more, talk less, say more,
hate less, love more and all good things will be yours.
-Swedish proverb

Non-caloric nutrients:

Non-calorie-containing nutrients include: vitamins, minerals, antioxidants, non-nutritive sweeteners and non-digestible fibers. Many non-caloric nutrients are required and we will literally die if we do not consume an adequate amount. We are all aware, for example of the result of Vitamin C deficiency – scurvy – a severely debilitating condition. We are less aware of what can happen if we have a deficient intake of zinc or Vitamin E, because the results may be less obvious or debilitating but still can have a significant impact on our health.

When we eat a variety of different foods, we are more likely to get a balance of vitamins and minerals in our diet. This is one of the risks of the restrictive diets, where certain foods or classes of foods are excluded from the diet. Those foods contain nutrients that are beneficial and by restricting what we eat, it becomes more difficult to get an adequate amount of the required nutrients. The resulting imbalance is likely more harmful than the small benefit gained from excluding these foods.

Dietary Fibers

Dietary fibers are carbohydrates of a special kind – these fibers are not digested in the stomach allowing them to pass intact into the intestines, where there are bacteria with the ability to digest them. There are many kinds of dietary fibers, some soluble in water and some insoluble. All are beneficial to human digestion and health by feeding intestinal bacteria and by increasing the viscosity of food in the intestine, slowing absorption of nutrients across the intestinal wall.

Some functional dietary fibers and where to find them include:

- Inulin: found in wheat, chicory root and artichokes
- Beta Glucan: found in oat bran, barley bran and yeast cell walls. This is the one of the best fibers to take, because not only is it good food for your bacteria, but it improves insulin sensitivity, and it acts as an immune modulator, meaning it enhances immune function when too low and moderates it when too high[23]. Recommended intake of beta glucan is 0.5 to 1 gram per day, easily gotten from oat bran cereal.
- Cellulose: found in wood fiber, cottonseed fiber, oat fiber, soy fiber, wheat fiber
- Polydextrose: produced by fermentation. As the name suggests, it is a polymer of glucose.
- Pectin: found in fruits especially in the skin of apples, oranges, grapefruit
- Psyllium husk: the husk from a psyllium seed. It is over 80% fiber, comes in a flake or powder form, has a pleasant, grainy flavor, easily mixes in water. Just don't try to bake with it – it absorbs so much water that it will ruin the texture of a batter or dough! I find psyllium to be one of the easiest fibers to incorporate into my diet, with lots of benefits and minimal digestive distress.
- Wheat bran: found in whole wheat products
- Resistant starch: found in baked products. I find it to be one of the easiest fibers to incorporate into my diet, with minimal negative impact.
- Gums: there are many kinds of gums used in food including: agar, acacia, guar, xanthan and carrageenan (yes, gums are often fibers, meaning they are not digested until the bacteria get to them in our intestines – and they are good!)

Adding fiber to your diet can be as simple as eating more vegetables like asparagus, kale, collards, brussels sprouts, or broccoli. Or more grains like whole wheat bread and oat bran. Or walnuts, cocoa powder, and cinnamon. Or taking supplements like psyllium. Start out low and increase your fiber intake slowly. Too much fiber, especially one that your digestive system is not capable of handling, can cause significant intestinal distress, including bloating, flatulence, sour stool, diarrhea, and anal leakage. Not a pretty picture. Go slowly and if you experience distress, stop and try a different fiber. I find the easiest to handle are psyllium, resistant starch (in bread), oat bran, wheat bran, cellulose, polydextrose and pectin. Beano® is a dietary supplement that contains enzymes to help digest fiber and can prevent flatulence and bloating. This can be especially useful when you will be eating some new foods, for example when traveling. I find that taking it for a few days is often enough. And once your microbiome catches up, you won't need it until the next change in diet.

Most of us, today are not ingesting sufficient amounts of dietary fiber to keep our intestinal bacteria healthy. The University of Arizona Cooperative Extension estimates that Americans consume about 11 grams of fiber per day, less than half of the 25 gram Recommended Daily Value set by the government for adults and children older than age four. The USDA Dietary Guidelines for Americans published in 2015 increased the recommended intake to 32 grams per day. I have seen recommendations ranging up to 100 grams per day. From my observations on my own diet, the magic number is 50 grams per day. There are many reasons why we under-consume fiber. Most people avoid eating the foods or parts of foods that are high in fiber. When we eat an apple or potato, we often remove the skin, which is where most of the fiber is located. The same is true of an orange or grapefruit. Admittedly, eating the peel of an orange is a bit difficult, but that is where most of the pectin and fiber are located. There is no fiber in meat, fish, eggs or any animal product. Only plants can make sugar and fiber. The fact remains that it is difficult to eat a diet with 50 grams of dietary fiber per day. There simply don't exist enough foods that are convenient to eat with sufficient fiber content to make it possible. We need to work on this.

Dietary fiber in the diet has many benefits including:

- Feeding the bacteria in our intestines
- Increasing the number and diversity of bacteria in the intestine, allowing them to colonize and form a layer of live bacterial cells on the surface of the intestine
- Creating a layer of mucous to coat the inside of the intestine
- Improving the balance of bacteria in the intestines
- Producing short chain fatty acids as a waste product of bacterial growth, reducing the pH of the intestine wall, making it more resistant to pathogenic infection
- Reducing the permeability of the intestine wall, preventing leaky gut syndrome which allows undigested food to enter the bloodstream where it can cause an allergic or immune response
- Increasing the viscosity of the food in the intestine, slowing down absorption of glucose into the blood stream, reducing the size of glucose spikes, improving blood glucose control, putting less stress on the system, preventing beta cell fatigue, preventing insulin resistance and eventually diabetes
- Producing short chain fatty acids that are absorbed into the bloodstream, improving the circulation of high melting point fatty materials such as LDL, VLDL, saturated fats and cholesterol, reducing the risk of heart disease
- Reducing blood pressure

When we increase the amount of fiber in our diet, magical things will start to happen. Things like losing weight and body fat, or improvements in blood chemistry, better control of blood glucose, reduced morning blood glucose fasting level, and a reduction in blood pressure.[24] It is best to measure and keep track of your blood glucose and blood pressure as you move to increase fiber in your diet, to enable you to learn how to manage the change well. Blood glucose levels below 75 for extended periods can make you dizzy or faint. And blood pressure, if it drops too low, can also be an issue. We want these changes to happen, but need to give our bodies time to adjust and manage properly. Measure and track.

We urgently need to get dietary fiber back into our diets at sufficient levels to solve the diseases of the Metabolic Syndrome, including diabetes.

Glycemic Index

The Glycemic Index (GI) is a measure of how the level of glucose in our bloodstream changes after eating a specific amount (usually 100 grams) of a food. It is a measure of how quickly the food is digested and absorbed into the bloodstream. Foods that are composed of high levels of sugar, or starch that is readily converted into glucose, are quickly absorbed directly into the bloodstream. The result is a rapid and sharp rise in blood glucose and insulin level in response. Pure sucrose is used calibrate the scale, has a GI of 100. Carbs that are complex, take more time to break down to release the sugars, and have GI values that are lower. Fiber, for example, is digested very slowly in the intestines and has a GI of near zero. The concept behind using the GI value in deciding what to eat is to avoid foods with high GI and eat more foods with low GI values, in order to limit the extent to which blood glucose rises after eating a meal. This is a good goal, as this will make it easier for the body to manage and avoid unhealthy, high levels of blood glucose. As usual, it is more complicated than that and foods cannot be effectively reduced to a number.

There are some problems with the GI value, starting with the way GI is determined. 100 grams of a pure foods is fed to people who have been fasting overnight. The test is to monitor how high their blood glucose level rises after eating 100 grams of the pure food. We seldom eat pure foods in isolation. The presence of other foods in the meal will change the way that the carbs in the food break down and therefore the GI of the food. Some other factors that will also have an impact are: fat content, how much is eaten, protein, fiber, how much water is taken with the food, how well we chew it, the temperature of the food, the condition of our digestive system, how ripe a fruit or vegetable is, and many others. This makes GI, by itself, an unreliable indicator.

The GI can help us identify which foods contain higher levels of readily digestible starches or free sugars that can be absorbed quickly into the bloodstream, potentially causing a spike in blood glucose levels. Eating these foods along with other foods, especially those that have low GI, will slow down the release and absorption of sugar and can reduce the glucose spike. Fats in the meal will slow down the digestion of starches. For example; butter on bread or toast will slow down the release of sugars and reduce the GI. Fiber in the diet will slow down absorption of sugar in the intestines. GI is a simple model for how quickly a food is converted into sugar, but in most cases, it is too simple.

Glycemic Load expands the concept of GI to take into account how much food is eaten and what foods are eaten in a meal to estimate the total glycemic response of the meal. This is better, but still there are lots of variables that are not accounted for. The best advice is to consider GI as a guide when selecting foods to eat but keep in mind the limitations.

In general, foods that are high in GI will cause a larger spike in blood glucose. However; it is more complicated than that. We can turn the complication around into an advantage, by learning how our body reacts to various combinations of foods. A great way to learn which foods or meals to avoid and which ones to eat more often, is to test our blood glucose. We can make a game of it, seeing who can design the meal with the lowest or no impact on blood glucose. Here is how the game is played:

1. Select a meal, where we combine different foods, with the purpose of minimizing the blood glucose spike.

2. Wait without eating anything for at least three hours, so that our blood glucose is at baseline. Measure it. Let's say we get 103.

3. Eat a reasonable amount of the meal. The amount we eat will impact the effect, usually more food causes a higher blood glucose spike. The idea here is to assess the impact of food as we would eat it and in the amount that we would normally eat. In the standard GI test, 100 grams of a food are consumed, but we usually don't eat foods alone, so it will be more natural and meaningful for us to prepare and eat the food as we normally would. For example: if we want to test how our body reacts to whole grain rice, cook it up as we normally would and then add the other ingredients that we want, such as salt, butter, olive oil, meat, veggies, etc., and eat it the combination as a meal.

4. Test blood glucose fifteen minutes after eating, and then every fifteen minutes until blood glucose returns to baseline.

5. In some cases, the level will spike up quickly and then drop again quickly, going down below the baseline, even plunging below 80. These are the foods we want to avoid or at least eat less of.

6. In other cases, the level will rise slowly and then just as slowly go back down to baseline. These are foods that our body can tolerate. We can include these in our diet in moderation.

7. In other cases, the level will not change at all. It just stays flat with no rise or decline. These are foods that our bodies can manage easily. We want to eat these more often.

8. Then for fun, try mixing the foods to create meals and see how it works. The goal is to design meals that have minimal impact on your blood glucose levels. This will reduce the stress on the blood glucose control system and allow our body to rest and recover from the barrage of glucose spikes experienced in the past.

9. Foods eaten alone will usually spike blood glucose more than when eaten in combination, especially if the other foods do not spike it. This is why the glycemic index is not very useful. Fats and oils, proteins and fiber are good for this. Rice is a good test example, as it is high in carbs and not high enough in protein, fiber or fat to moderate the digestion and rapid absorption of sugar into the bloodstream. Therefore, eating rice can spike our blood glucose to unhealthy levels. We can avoid eating rice or find a way to eat it in a way that allows our body to process it safely. First, eat less. It is much easier for our body to deal with a few tablespoons of any food than a heaping portion. And, eat it with other foods that contain fat, fiber and protein. Putting butter or oil on the rice will help. Mixing in some chia seeds or pine nuts will add protein, fat and fiber. Get in the habit of adding nuts to recipes, as they are high in protein, fiber and fat, and will moderate glucose absorption, in addition to other health benefits. All good.[25]

10. Drinking while eating will usually spike blood glucose more quickly, therefore avoid drinking a lot during a meal. Wait thirty minutes, then drink that beer, or sip it slowly while eating. Wine is fine during a meal, as the amount of liquid is low.

11. Making the food more viscous will decrease the rate of sugar absorption. We can do this by drinking a psyllium shake with a food that is high in carbs. The recipe is in Appendix 6. We can add chia seeds to a food to add viscosity and fat. That will slow the absorption of sugar. I drink a psyllium shake before eating a few fresh peaches from a tree in my yard and my blood glucose barely budges. Drinking a psyllium shake before eating a meal can also be a good practice, with several benefits: it will increase the viscosity of the food, slowing sugar absorption; it will feed the bacteria in the intestines; it will fill us up a bit, allowing us to eat less. All good.

Some foods have little or no impact on blood glucose, and are useful to eat alone or in combination with the high glycemic index foods to help moderate the absorption of sugar into the bloodstream. Some good examples include:

- Sunflower seeds
- Nuts – especially pistachio nuts because they are high in fiber
- Psyllium shakes
- Chia seeds
- Protein shakes (keep the sugar below 5 grams)
- Chocolate (85% cocoa or higher)
- Artichoke hearts (a cup is only 114 calories and has 14 grams of fiber, mostly inulin)
- Beer – in fact most alcoholic drinks, that are low in sugar, and consumed in moderation, will have no impact

And remember, that eating more of any food will result in a higher spike in blood glucose. Just eating less of that food will reduce the spike.

I suggested making it a game. The game we want to play is figuring out how to incorporate the foods we love or want in our diet, in a manner that allows our bodies to competently manage blood glucose levels. For example: Oat bran cereal has more beta glucan than any other food. I want it in my diet, but it is also high in carbs and will spike blood glucose levels if eaten alone. Combining oat bran with other ingredients can reduce the GI and the blood glucose spike. Cocoa and cinnamon are reported to improve control of blood glucose – let's add those. Fat will slow down the absorption of the sugars into the bloodstream – let's add some. Viscosity will help slow down the absorption of sugar – let's add chia seeds. And so on, until we find a way to make it possible to eat oat bran and not worry about blood glucose. See the recipe in Appendix 4. This is a game we play for keeps – for our life. Game on!

Supplements

A combination of different foods will usually provide a mix of nutrients to meet our needs. The exceptions to this are Vitamin E, Vitamin C and magnesium. I said that there wasn't a pill that will help you to extend your healthy life. I lied a little. There are actually several pills that you should consider taking to improve your health.

Supplements are a controversial subject, but until we find foods that we will eat enough of to provide the benefits we are looking for, supplements are worth taking. One benefit of a supplement is that it has been standardized to deliver a specific amount of a nutrient or active ingredient. We don't have that kind of control over the foods we eat. Foods vary in freshness, cooking methods, amount consumed, absorption rate, etc. Nutrients and active ingredients may not be active or bioavailable in the food we eat. Turmeric is a good example. Turmeric spice contains the active ingredient curcumin, but the bioavailability varies greatly. The supplement is processed to assure that the curcumin is bioavailable and absorbable by the body. The supplement is usually validated, reliable and convenient – check them out to confirm.

Here are some supplements for you to consider taking every day:

- Vitamin D – most of us are deficient in Vitamin D because we don't get enough sun. Vitamin D has been found to be very important in preventing cancer. I take 6,000 IU twice a day. Next time you have a blood test, ask for Vitamin D to be included so that you can assess if you are getting enough. You want to be at the top end of the 30-100 ng/ml range that the medical profession identifies as 'normal'. And keep in mind that the FDA Recommended Daily Value is based on disease prevention, meaning the amount you need to take so that you don't develop a disease due to insufficient intake. We don't want to be there. We want to take an adequate amount for optimal health and of course disease prevention. That is a much higher amount. Vitamin D is not toxic until very high intakes on the order of 40,000 to 100,000 IU per day according to the Mayo Clinic, so the risk of overconsumption is very low.

- Curcumin – select a bioactive form either in pill or liquid liposomal dispersion. It is a powerful antioxidant and helps to reduce inflammation. This has to be one of the best finds for life extension ever. There are no known negative side effects to curcumin. The impact is all good. It is also called turmeric spice. Using the spice in cooking is great for flavor, fiber and antioxidants, but the absorption of the antioxidant from the spice is limited, which is why it's important to get the bioactive form.

- Antioxidants – necessary to combat oxidative stress. Antioxidants react with free radicals in the body to protect against damage due to oxidation. Grapeseed extract is a good one. Dr. Life is marketing an herbal blend that is more active than typical antioxidants[4]. Antioxidants also reduce inflammation. You can include some good antioxidants such as turmeric, cinnamon and cocoa in your cooking. These are also good sources of dietary fiber.

- Charcoal powder – this is a very finely ground powdered, activated, pure charcoal. It has a tremendous surface area because the particles are so small, making it highly active for absorbing toxins from food in the intestines. All food contains toxins, most of them naturally occurring in the plant as a defense mechanism against being eaten. We and the plants have been playing a game of one-ups-man-ship forever. They create a new toxin; we develop an antidote or way to detoxify it. Our body is very good at this, but wouldn't complain if we gave it a little help. Charcoal powder is a way to help. It doesn't take much – about a gram or two a day is plenty. Don't get scared, as it will turn your poop a deep, elegant black color. That's about all you will notice. But it will help improve your intestinal function and intestinal microbiome. It is in the All-In Biome Balance ™ Bagel. Eating one of these bagels each day will give you plenty of charcoal. Or you can add it to your psyllium shake or even oat bran cereal if you are daring.

- Melatonin – a good antioxidant to reduce inflammation and a great sleep aid. Even if you are sleeping adequately, you will notice a difference. Take ten to twenty five mg of melatonin right before going to sleep.

- Multivitamin – just to be sure that you're not missing anything important.

- Omega-3 fish oil – the only good source of required Eicosapentanaenoic acid (0.25 grams per day), which we need for our brain. The other required fats are linoleic acid (10 grams a day required, which we can get from 1 tablespoon of walnut or grapeseed oil) and linolenic acid (2 grams a day required, which we can get from a teaspoon of flaxseed oil). Our bodies cannot make these oils and also cannot store them, so it is important that they are part of our diet. We can make flaxseed or grapeseed oil part of our diet every day by using these oils on salads or in our cooking. Fish oils are more difficult due to their extreme sensitivity to oxidation. And you probably don't want to eat salmon or fish every day. The krill oil supplement is the best fish oil.

- Collagen (types I, II and III) – necessary for healthy joints, skin, nails and intestines. We don't get enough collagen in the meat we eat today, because we eat almost exclusively muscle meats, avoiding cartilage and organ meats, which are high in collagen. When you start taking collagen daily, you will be amazed at the impact on your skin and nails. These are the most visible places where collagen is important. Your intestines are also composed of collagen protein, so as your nails improve, your intestines are also improving. That is where we want to be.

- Prebiotic beneficial bacteria – spore-based ones such as Thrive® are best as they survive stomach acids and become active in the intestine, where needed. The foods we eat today are too sterile. Most have been treated with an antimicrobial spray or processed to reduce or eliminate pathogenic bacteria. That sounds like a good thing, as it prevents illness due to contaminated food. However; these treatments also reduce or eliminate the good bacteria that our digestive system needs to function properly. I personally think that FDA is on the wrong path, trying to make food sterile. Food is not sterile, is not meant to be sterile and will never be sterile unless we kill everything. That will not be good for anyone. Rather, we need to propagate and nurture a healthy bacterial microbiome in our intestines in order to enhance our immune systems and protect us from the few pathogenic bacteria we are going to ingest, no matter how hard FDA tries to prevent it. If we don't have enough bacteria in our intestines and we don't feed them properly so that they propagate and dominate, then pathogenic bacteria will find a hospitable environment and cause illness. There is a constant battle going on in our intestines between different kinds of bacteria. We want assure a healthy quantity and balance of bacteria, that make the intestines inhospitable to pathogenic bacteria.
- Psyllium fiber – two tablespoons in a glass of water once a day works wonders for our digestive system, not to mention the good it does for our bathroom visits! We don't get enough fiber in the foods we eat. We tend to avoid high fiber foods such as kale, collards, wheat bran, oat bran, etc. The result is that the bacteria in our intestines are undernourished. This means that the quantity and quality of the bacteria in our intestines is suboptimal. Getting bacteria into our intestines is only half the fight. Once there, we must feed them to keep them healthy. When the bacteria are there and fed well on

dietary fiber, they produce short chain fatty acids as a waste product (yes, we are talking about their poop!). These are predominantly propionic acid and butyric acid and have many health benefits.[26] They reduce the pH in the vicinity of the intestinal wall where the bacteria are colonizing. This protects the intestinal wall from invasion by pathogenic or illness-causing bacteria, which cannot tolerate the low pH. And these short chain fatty acids are absorbed into the bloodstream where they help keep fats and cholesterol moving and not clogging.

- Magnesium — if you experience leg cramps, especially common at night, you may be deficient in magnesium. Magnesium can be taken as a pill, a spray or even as an Epsom salt soak.

Hypochondria is the only disease I haven't got.
-Anonymous

CHAPTER 4

THE DIGESTION PROCESS

Digestion is the process of breaking down the food we eat into a form that is capable of being absorbed across the intestinal wall into the bloodstream, delivering the nutrients to our organs and cells. Digestion begins in the mouth, where the food is masticated to reduce the size of the pieces. Mastication makes it possible for us to swallow the food, increases the available surface area and mixes the food with water and amylase enzymes supplied by saliva in our mouths. After swallowing, the food is delivered via the esophagus into the stomach, where the food is mixed with more enzymes and acid. Enzymes are specialized proteins, some of which are present in the foods we eat, others are secreted into our stomachs, and still more are produced by bacteria in our digestive system. These enzymes include amylases that breaks down starch into sugar, lipases that breaks down fats and oils into fatty acids and glycerin, and proteases that break down protein into amino acids. Lysozyme is a very powerful enzyme present inside the cells of the food we eat that is released when the cells are ruptured during the digestion process. These enzymes include those that can break down dietary fibers, bran and even to some extent cellulose. Bacteria in the human gut can only partially digest cellulose fiber and therefore, for us, cellulose is not an efficient food source.

Intestines

Most of the work of digestion and absorption of food occurs in the intestines. It is a complex and fascinating structure that winds through our belly, measuring over thirty feet in length. It is flexible and irregular in shape, but essentially it is a pipe through which food materials travel. Partially digested food comes in one end, from the stomach and travels through the small intestine until it is passed into the large intestine. It takes one to three days for the food to complete the journey. As the food moves along, the enzymes and acid from the mouth and stomach are augmented by enzymes excreted by bacteria that colonize the walls of the intestine. These bacteria, collectively, are called our microbiome. Our microbiome not only influences how we digest food, but when it is unbalanced, has negative impacts on the entire body that include obesity, the diseases of the Metabolic Syndrome, how our bodies look and even how we behave. A fascinating article on the importance of our humble gut bacteria is "Feeding the brain and nurturing the mind: Linking nutrition and the gut microbiota to brain development", by Manu S. Goyal, et. al.[27, 28] We will discuss the microbiome in more detail and how our failure to keep it healthy leads to disease.

In the intestines, excess water is removed from the digesting food and absorbed. Dietary fibers are broken down and some of the sugar and small chain fatty acids produced are absorbed into the bloodstream. The dietary fiber present in our food, serves as a food source for the bacteria and when we don't eat enough fiber, these bacteria are undernourished, underactive or even cause damage by consuming the mucosal wall of the intestine, resulting in a leaky gut that allows undigested food materials into the bloodstream, with many bad consequences. The microbiome in our intestines can be changed by what we eat, both in quantity and balance. If we change our diet by eating a food we haven't eaten in a while, the microbiome may not be capable of providing the right enzymes to digest this food and the result can be some intestinal distress. For example, if a person who has been eating a vegetarian diet for some time eats meat, they may experience some digestive distress as their microbiome will respond negatively to the new food. Another example is found in people who remove gluten from their diets for some time and then eat a slice of bread. They feel some distress and conclude that the gluten is really bad for them, when their microbiome is reacting badly to a food it hasn't seen in a while and for which it is not prepared. Similarly, eating a big serving of beans, when you haven't eaten beans on a regular basis, will result in severe flatulence and discomfort. The problem isn't the beans, but rather that your microbiome was unprepared for the quantity or type of beans you ingested.

It is critically important to our health that sugars in food are absorbed slowly, giving the body time to metabolize the glucose, to properly process and store the excess as glycogen and to safely convert fructose into glucose. These factors, plus the fact that the glucose is entering the blood slowly, reduce the amount of glucose in the blood at a given time and decrease the size of the spike in blood glucose level. Remember that the main cause of diabetes and failure to control blood glucose is the repeated presence of high levels of glucose that stress and damage the control system. Sugar absorption through the intestinal wall and into the bloodstream is mediated by several factors. The first line of defense against rapid sugar absorption is having sufficient bacteria in the intestines. The bacteria colonize the surface of the intestinal wall, forming an additional layer that traps mucous and acts as a barrier to slow down the absorption of glucose.[29]

Another factor that slows down the absorption of glucose into the bloodstream, and is critical in the prevention of diabetes, is the presence of fiber in food. Not only does the fiber feed the intestinal bacteria, but it absorbs water and increases the viscosity of the food material as it passes through the intestine. This slows down the absorption of glucose through the intestinal wall into the bloodstream. It gives the bacteria in the intestine more time to ferment the glucose and convert it into good materials like short chain fatty acids. As important as low sugar consumption is in preventing diabetes and the other diseases of the

Metabolic Syndrome, the real underlying cause is insufficient dietary fiber. This lack of dietary fiber has depleted the microbiome in our intestines, resulting in leaky intestines that allow undigested proteins to enter the bloodstream, causing autoimmune diseases. Low fiber levels in the intestines allow sugar to enter the bloodstream rapidly causing damaging blood glucose spikes, result in a lack of short chain fatty acids, which make the intestine more susceptible to pathogenic bacterial infections, and if that isn't enough, the lack of short chain fatty acids in our blood results in poor ability to manage high melting point fatty materials, resulting in circulatory damage and heart disease. Returning dietary fiber to the diet is the key to resolving all of these diseases.

When we consider our intestines, we can see how the three factors of diet, activity and microbiome are connected. Diet comprises what we put into the digestive system, how much and when. Activity effects the muscles that push and squeeze the food materials while in the digestive system, resulting in mixing, size reduction, residence time, water removal and many other benefits. A lack of sufficient physical activity results in poor digestion. Humans were designed to walk and be far more active than we are today. Our intestines suffer because of our inactivity and poor abdominal muscle tone. We don't need to be professional athletes, or have a 'six-pack' abdomen, but rather just keep active to help out our intestines. The intestinal microbiome digests food and keeps the intestinal wall healthy and efficient at keeping undigested food inside the intestine where it belongs and not in the bloodstream where it can cause severe damage. Resolving the Metabolic Syndrome requires restoring balance to these three. And remember, that I'm a 'Darm' Mann (from Darmstadt – intestine city) and so are you!

Microbiome

The bacteria in or on our body are collectively called the microbiome. The intestines are home to thousands of different kinds of bacteria, but so are the skin, mouth, vagina and other places. It is estimated that there are up to one hundred trillion bacteria making up our microbiome, weighing about five pounds. There is a natural balance of the types and number of bacteria that is a result of what we feed them and how we treat them. When the balance of bacteria in the intestines is compromised, some types of bacteria can get out of control, while others may be depleted. It is not so much that some bacteria are good and others are bad, excepting pathogenic bacteria of course, but many different types are required in proper balance for good health. The balance can be altered by taking antibiotics, eating foods with powerful emulsifiers, eating too much sugar, eating too little fiber, eating a restricted diet, and more. These bacteria protect the intestine from pathogenic microorganisms and determine how the intestines digest the foods we eat.

Plants produce a class of proteins called lectins that are anti-nutritive factors, designed to discourage insects and animals from eating the plant. There are hundreds of such proteins in almost all plants, especially in the seeds[30]. Beans, especially soybeans and fava beans, contain trypsin inhibitor, as an example, that prevents digestion of the bean proteins. An animal or insect that eats the bean will have severe digestive distress. This includes humans. The good news is that cooking denatures and detoxifies most of the lectin, so we have learned to cook beans. Wheat gluten is another lectin protein. After cooking, the second line of defense against these proteins is in our intestine. The lectin proteins bind to the mucous in the intestine. The bacteria in the mucous produce enzymes that can break down the lectins, turning them into harmless amino acids. When the mucous layer and the bacteria in it are in good condition and balance, we are protected from the lectin proteins produced by plants. And cooking helps too!

Leaky Gut Syndrome

The wall of the intestine is partially porous, in order to allow only digested food material to pass through and enter into the bloodstream. The wall consists of a several layers: a cell membrane, live bacteria and a coating of mucous, that together produce a barrier that prevents undigested particles of food from passing through. When the layer of colonizing bacteria and mucous is damaged or missing, as can happen when we take antibiotics, the wall of the intestine allows partially digested food to pass into the bloodstream. This is called leaky gut syndrome. These partially digested food materials, include fats or oils (as opposed to fatty acids), polypeptides (as opposed to amino acids) or multi-unit starches (as opposed to sugar), don't belong in our bloodstream and will cause problems there. The purpose of digestion is to break down food into fatty acids, sugar and amino acids. When undigested fats or oils enter the bloodstream, the result is irritation to the walls of the arteries, which causes a defense response where a layer of protective plaque is applied on the artery lining. As this process repeats itself, the successive layers of plaque accumulate to eventually block the artery – causing arterial failure and heart disease. Note that the root cause of plaque buildup is not that we ate fat, the wrong kind of fat or even too much fat. The root cause is the presence of undigested fats and oils in the bloodstream, where they do not belong. Polypeptides that enter the bloodstream will be detected by the immune systems as foreign objects to be attacked and removed. When this response is severe, it can result in an allergic or autoimmune reaction. The foreign polypeptide may have the same amino acid sequence as a polypeptide that is present somewhere else in our bodies, for example the cartilage in our joints. When our immune system is sensitized to attack this particular polypeptide by partially digested food that gets into our bloodstream, the same immune response can result in an attack on the cartilage in our joints. The immune system cannot differentiate between the foreign material and the material that is present in our body, so it attacks the material in our body as well. This is possibly how arthritis and other autoimmune diseases like Sclera-Derma and allergies may be caused. Again, please note that the root cause of these diseases is not that we ate protein, the wrong kind of protein or even too much protein, but the presence of undigested protein in the bloodstream, where it doesn't belong. The leaky gut is the issue that we must correct via diet and exercise.

The healthy intestinal wall is composed of living cells, bacteria and finally mucous. The purpose of this multi-layered wall is to contain undigested food materials inside the intestine, until adequate digestion occurs, at which point the fully digested food molecules are small enough to pass through the semi-permeable intestinal wall and enter the bloodstream. The size of the molecule determines which pass and which are retained inside the intestine for further digestion. It is a critical function of the intestinal wall to protect the body from exposure to potentially harmful material. The intestinal wall is literally the 'skin' inside our bodies, and like the skin that covers our bodies, it acts as a barrier between the outside world and our inner organs. With the intestines located inside of our bodies, it may be difficult to see them as a barrier to the outside world, but all of the food and water that we ingest from the outside world must pass through our intestines in order to enter the body. The intestine acts as a screen, keeping potentially harmful materials out of the body, while allowing beneficial nutrients into the body. Differentiating between the good and the bad is not so easy. We depend on a healthy intestine to do that and suffer when the intestine is unhealthy.

Recent research on diets that are deficient in dietary fiber confirm not only the benefits of fiber on the health of the bacteria in our intestines, but go far further. A study by a group at the Luxembourg Institute of Health led by Mahesh S. Desai[31] has found that when the diet is deficient in fiber, the bacteria in our intestines are deprived of nutrients and instead metabolize the mucous layer inside the intestine wall. The title of their paper says it all: *"A Dietary Fiber-Deprived Gut Microbiota Degrades the Colonic Mucous Barrier and Enhances Pathogen Susceptibility"*. This degradation by the starved bacteria, creates holes in the mucous layer, causing a leaky gut. This is a shocking and critical finding with huge health consequences related to all the diseases of the Metabolic Syndrome. This is the smoking gun that we have been looking for.

When we don't have enough fiber in our diet, the bacteria that colonize the intestinal wall, do not have sufficient food and instead they digest the mucosal layer itself, making holes in the layer. This is very bad and the cause of a long list of negative health impacts, including:

- The mucosal layer protects the wall of the intestine from damage due to irritating materials in the food. When the intestinal wall is exposed, the acids and enzymes that digest the food will also attack the intestinal wall. And, it's a fact that even 'natural' food contains toxins and irritants. Do you like hot sauce or spices? When the intestine is unprotected, these materials can cause damage, irritation and inflammation. The result can be colitis or irritable bowel syndrome (IBS).
- The mucosal layer provides a home for bacteria. When they are fed adequate amounts of fiber, these bacteria produce small chain fatty acids like acetic acid, butyric acid and propionic acid that decrease the pH of the mucosal layer, which makes it inhospitable to pathogenic bacteria like Listeria, Salmonella and E. coli. Viral particles in the food will have a more difficult time attaching to the wall of the intestine when the mucosal layer is intact. The result of a compromised mucosal layer is that we get sick more often.
- The mucous lining the healthy intestine is a lubricant, allowing food material inside to flow easily as it digests. This lubrication will also be beneficial when it's time for the fully digested and dewatered material to exit the body.
- The bacteria in the intestine produce vitamins that are released into the digesting food and absorbed through the intestinal wall and into the bloodstream. The bacteria in the intestine literally feed us. When our diet contains too

little fiber, the bacteria starve, their number or balance are compromised, and we starve!

- The mucosal layer slows down the rate of absorption of nutrients into the bloodstream. The result, when the layer is intact, is that nutrients are absorbed slowly over a longer period of time than when the layer is missing or compromised. Slow absorption allows the systems of the body that manage nutrients, like glucose, more time to respond. When glucose from a meal is absorbed too quickly, the result is a sharp spike in blood glucose level that in turn spikes insulin. Too much insulin production causes the liver, brain and muscles to become insulin resistant, eventually causing diabetes. Too much insulin production causes the beta cells in the pancreas to eventually fatigue and fail to produce sufficient insulin, eventually resulting in diabetes. Moderating the rate of absorption of nutrients, especially glucose across the intestinal wall is a critical to preventing diabetes.

- The mucosal layer with embedded bacteria binds and breaks down natural toxins in food such as lectins, protecting us from the harmful effects of these anti-nutritive proteins.

- The holes in the mucosal layer create a leaky gut. The intestinal wall is a barrier between the undigested food inside the intestine and the bloodstream. Food is supposed to be digested inside the intestine and absorbed across the intestinal wall only when broken down into simple sugars, amino acids and fatty acids. When undigested or partially digested protein polymers are able to pass through the leaky gut into the bloodstream, the immune system detects them as foreign materials, is sensitized, produces antibodies and destroys the foreign protein. This is how the immune system operates. The problem is when the sequence of amino acids in the foreign food protein happens to match the amino acid sequence of a tissue inside the body, the immune system cannot tell the difference. The sensitized immune system will search out proteins with that specific amino acid sequence wherever they may be in the body. If that protein is in the knuckles or joints, the result is arthritis. If in the skin, the result is scleroderma or psoriasis. If the protein is in the beta cells of the pancreas that produce insulin, the result is type I diabetes.

- Our bodies are a holism – all parts connected, all parts contributing, all parts important. A leaky gut is the first step in a chain of harmful events that leads to diabetes, getting sick more often from the flu and food poisoning, obesity, allergic reactions to food, autoimmune diseases, intestinal disorders like IBS and colitis, high blood pressure, heart disease, cancer and more. Fixing our intestines should be our number one priority.

Unfortunately, there are many ways to damage the healthy intestinal wall:

- Taking antibiotics kills the bacteria that colonize and coat the surface of the wall, with numerous bad consequences. We should only take antibiotics when necessary to fight an infection. Afterwards, we need to pay special attention to restoring the bacteria in our intestines. In the next section, please read on how to do that.
- Eating a diet that is low in dietary fiber fails to provide the food that the bacteria need to live and grow in sufficient number.
- Eating a diet that is high in sugar changes the balance of bacteria in the intestine, allowing some to proliferate, while others decline. The balance of many different kinds

of bacteria are beneficial to digestion, nutrition, the immune system, resistance to infection and much more.

- Eating a diet that contains strong emulsifying agents. Emulsifiers are materials that stabilize tiny droplets of fats and oils that can then be suspended in water, forming a stable emulsion. Many foods are emulsified and there are many kinds of emulsifiers. There are natural emulsifiers including milk proteins, egg lecithin, soybean lecithin, and these are strong enough to form stable food emulsions like ice cream and milk, but not strong enough to act as detergents. There are synthetic emulsifiers, such as polysorbate 60, that are much stronger and are able to act as detergents. This is an important difference, because the detergent action of synthetic emulsifiers is capable of damaging the cell wall of bacteria. Plants and animals have cell walls based on cellulose and lipoproteins, respectively. This is why detergents do not harm our skin or plants. But bacterial cell walls are mostly made of fat and can be disrupted by a detergent. This is how soaps and detergents clean our dirty hands and also act as sanitizers, killing bacteria. This is all good for hands and kitchen counter tops. The problem comes when these strong emulsifiers are in food that ends up inside of our intestines, where they can disrupt the cell walls of bacteria, causing damage to our microbiome.

There are ways for us to maintain or recover the healthy intestine, especially:

- Eating foods that contain fiber, such as whole grains, vegetables, fruits, spices and chocolate. Only plants can make fiber. We must feed our bacteria with fiber to keep them healthy. Indigestible fibers pass through our stomach and enter the intestine undigested. The bacteria digest the fibers and excrete small chain fatty acids as their waste product. Perfect! These fatty acids, mostly butyric acid and propionic acid, reduce the pH of the intestinal wall, making it inhospitable to pathogenic bacteria and are absorbed directly into the bloodstream, where they clean arteries.

- The 2015 USDA Dietary Guidelines for Americans recommends 25 and 38 grams per day of dietary fiber depending on sex and caloric intake. There is insufficient evidence to claim with certainty that this is enough fiber. I have found that for me, 50 grams a day is a good target level. We may have to learn how much is right for us individually. Start low and increase the level of fiber in your diet SLOWLY. If you eat too much fiber, your intestines will rebel and you will not be a happy camper. By adding fiber and slowly increasing the amount in your diet, you give the bacteria in your intestines time to adapt in quantity and type. Too much, too fast will overburden the ability of the bacteria to digest the fiber and cause distress including bloating, flatulence, and even pain. It has taken decades to train our digestive system to be what it is. Don't expect it to change overnight. Retraining the system will take several months.

- Take probiotics in moderation. Probiotics are concentrated doses of live bacteria. About 99% of the live bacteria that we ingest, will be killed in our stomach, but a pill that contains ten billion live bacteria can still deliver one hundred million live cells into the intestines. The best probiotics contain spores, which survive the stomach and enter the intestines intact ready to grow. Some are now advising against taking probiotics, claiming that we really don't know which bacteria are beneficial and by adding the wrong ones we could actually make things worse. We already have the bacteria that we need in our intestines, just not in the right balance, because of poor diet. Fixing the diet will allow the balance to improve and correct itself. That is a compelling argument.

- Eat foods that are fermented. These include yogurt (unsweetened), kefir, kombucha, sour kraut, fermented vegetables, and unpasteurized beer. The food we eat is too clean and free of bacteria. Even the lettuce we buy today has been ozone treated to reduce the risk of pathogenic bacteria. This is fine, except the good bacteria go the same way as the bad – dead. We benefit from a constant influx of good bacteria into our guts to keep the good guys in control and the bad ones under control. Even if the live bacteria in the yogurt or sauerkraut are mostly killed in the stomach, we still benefit from all the healthy fermentation byproducts such as short chain fatty acids. Eating fermented foods will favor the growth of good bacteria in the intestine and help reestablish or maintain the proper balance.

- Exercise!!! Our intestines need strong abdominal muscles to move the digesting food and waste products through in a reasonable time. The motion of the exercise helps too. Stomach crunches and sit-ups are ideal.
- Avoid antibiotics as much as possible. Avoid foods that contain synthetic emulsifiers and polyols.

There are some other diseases such as autism and schizophrenia that are now also hypothesized to be caused by the leaky condition of the gut. Dr. Natasha Campbell-McBride has written a book called *Gut Psychology Syndrome: Natural Treatment for Autism, Dyspraxia, A.D.D., Dyslexia, Depression, Schizophrenia* [32] in which she describes the horrible gut condition of people with these diseases and the work she has done to reverse it. We can learn a lot from her work and apply it to our own quest for a healthy intestine. If we want to extend our healthy life, we will need to learn.

The road to health is paved with good intestines!
-Dr. Sherry A. Rogers
In: Yafa, Stephen. "Grain of Truth." Penguin
Publishing Group, 2015-04-13. iBooks.

We have a lot to learn about our microbiome and the condition of our intestines. What we do know is that we have done a poor job of caring for our intestines through the use of antibiotics, poor diet and lack of exercise. If we want to extend our healthy lives, we need to learn how to nurture and care for our intestines, and cure our leaky gut.

Toilet Paper

Did you ever wonder why we are the only animal on the planet that needs to clean themselves after defecating? Do you think cavemen and women walked around with toilet paper or maybe they used leaves? Not likely. The answer is that we would not need to use toilet paper either, if our digestive systems were working properly. The answer is once again a combination of diet, activity and the microbiome.

It starts with what we eat. The component of food that is most responsible for our need to use toilet paper, is fiber. Fiber absorbs water in the intestine and acts as a bulking agent in the stool, increasing water-binding capacity, increasing mass and providing structure. All good features, but the real reason that fiber is so beneficial, is that it feeds our microbiome, which acts as a trap for mucous, a slippery, viscous fluid that is an effective lubricant. It is in saliva to lubricate food to help it pass cleanly and painlessly down the esophagus. It is also inside our intestines as a lubricant to help the food materials move along easily as they digest and transform from food particles to stool. Lubrication aids in the efficient movement, prevents constipation, prevents damage to the intestinal wall and reduces residence time in the digestive system. All good things.

The mucous that is present in a healthy gut due to the healthy bacterial layer has another benefit. It coats the surface of the stool as it passes through the intestine. When the stool exits through the anus, this layer of mucous acts as a lubricant so that the stool exits cleanly and easily. Another clue is how long do you spend on the toilet? When the stool is properly formed, and lubricated by mucous, it shouldn't take more than thirty seconds to do our business.

The stool is squeezed by the muscles in the abdominal wall, which is why activity is also important. Strong abdominal muscles, which are the result of exercise and activity can properly squeeze the intestines to form the stool, remove water and coat it with mucous. Weak abdominal muscles cannot do the job and the food and stool move slowly and inefficiently through the intestine, causing excessive residence time, excessive amounts of waste in the intestines, bloating, flatulence, pain and constipation. The best exercise for good intestinal function is the sit-up. Do at least ten sit-ups per day. Activity such as walking also keeps the food moving properly while it is in the intestines. If we are constipated or bloated, instead of taking medicine, consider activity level and of course, fiber intake.

Do you know where bad breath comes from? It often comes from what we eat, of course, but mostly it comes from our intestines. When our intestines are out of balance, we will notice it in our breath. There is research being done now to assess a person's health based on an analysis of their breath. This can work because the aromatic compounds in the breath come from other parts of the body, especially the intestines.

To summarize; when we have the following issues, there is an imbalance in our diet which is causing an imbalance in our intestinal microbiome, probably too little fiber or too much sugar, or both:

- Poop is smelly
- Poop sinks in water (it should float)
- Poop is sticky or tarry, making cleanup difficult
- Pooping hurts
- Poop is sour, maybe even burning or irritating your behind
- Poop is hard as a rock
- Pooping is explosive with lots of gas
- Poop is loose and not formed into units
- Poop is liquid and watery

These issues are not normal and we should not live with them. Something is wrong and we can fix it. The benefits will go far beyond our intestines. I hope this discussion wasn't too graphic, but it really is a serious issue and a good clue about balance or lack of balance in our diet, activity and microbiome. And, nothing feels as good as a good you know what!

CHAPTER 5

CONSTRUCTING A DIET

Dieting and Weight Management

First, let's differentiate between diet and dieting. Our diet is the sum of all the food and meals we eat. We all have a diet that is uniquely our own, based on the multitude of decisions we make every day about the food we eat. Our diet can be consistent or inconsistent depending on the choices we make. In contrast, 'Dieting' is the popular notion of modifying our diet to achieve some dietary goal, usually weight loss or health improvement. Dieting is often unsuccessful or only successful in the short term. We may achieve our weight reduction goal in the short term by dieting, but after the dieting is over, if we return to our original diet, then we should expect to go back to our original weight. This should be obvious, but most people see dieting only as a short-term practice to achieve a goal. This is faulty thinking. Unless we change our diet for the long term, we should not expect success from dieting. This is why our diet needs to be part of our lifestyle. If we are overweight or overeating, then we need to modify our diet and incorporate the changes into our lifestyle for long term success. We need to manage our diet and get beyond 'dieting'!

It is easier to change a man's religion than to change his diet.
-Margaret Mead

Portion control is the most important part of controlling our diet. When it comes to eating, size does matter! Most of us have no concept of what one hundred grams of avocado looks like. There are studies that show that people eat more when their plates are larger – so maybe it will help if we use a smaller plate. The best investment we can make (besides this book of course!) is to spend $50 on a small digital scale. There are some very nice units available in any good cooking supply store that will weigh up to 2000 grams. Use it to calibrate your eye by weighing the ingredients or components of your meals. This will help you to manage how much you eat and develop a diet that fits your personal preferences while achieving your dietary goals. Any food can be incorporated into a healthy diet with the proper portion control and balance with other foods.

As we have already discovered, taking in more calories than we need on a chronic basis over years, is the underlying root cause of the Metabolic Syndrome. We need to get control of how much we eat if we are going to be successful. Food very often becomes a surrogate for boredom and an antidote for stress. In addition, we eat by the clock and eat what is put before us, or what we think is appropriate. Buffets are often the worst because if people are allowed to eat all they want, most will eat more. We need to be aware of how much we are eating, pay attention and then choose thoughtfully, not in a reactionary or emotional manner. Eating is important business.

There are differing views on the frequency and timing of eating. Our bodies produce insulin in order to metabolize and control glucose, but insulin also regulates fat metabolism. Basically, our bodies only metabolize glucose when insulin levels are high and only metabolize fat when insulin levels are low. We want to design our diet so that our bodies are able to efficiently process the foods we eat while avoiding excessive blood glucose spikes that can lead to diabetes.

Have you ever watched a wild animal, like a deer or groundhog eat? Unfortunately, I get that opportunity too often as my desk overlooks the backyard, so I helplessly watch these critters graze on my trees, bushes and flower gardens! The interesting thing, is that they eat a variety of plants, and do not gorge themselves on just one, even when that one plant is available in surfeit. I have a long hedge of Wisteria, so in the spring there are a lot of tender Wisteria shoots available, and the deer stop and eat some. They could stand there all day and eat themselves full on just the Wisteria, if they chose to. But they don't. They eat a few here and a few there and then move on to the next tasty plants, which are usually my Purple Cone Flowers or Shasta Daisies! I believe they eat in this manner, not out of compassion for the plants, or me, but rather to get a variety of plants into their diet for nutritional purposes. In addition, almost all plants contain anti-nutritive ingredients or natural toxins designed to protect the plant from being eaten, and by eating a small amount of many different plants, the deer can avoid consuming a toxic overload of the anti-nutritive factor from any one plant. We can benefit by learning from the deer and doing the same. The concepts of balance and variety are critical to diet. Ideally we want our diet to provide a good balance of protein, carbs, fats, vitamins and minerals in proportion to what our bodies need, and the best way to do this is by consuming a wide variety of foods.

There are some excellent apps available today to help us keep track of what we eat and the nutrients contained. In an app called 'Bitesnap', we take a photo of our food, and the App is often able to identify the food and the nutritional content. If it fails, you can search for it or even add it. It is convenient, powerful and fun to use.

Food and Comfort

Who can deny the pleasure of eating a well-prepared meal with quality ingredients that complement in flavor, aroma, texture and appearance? Having enough to eat is satisfying and pleasurable as well. Food is a major source of pleasure in our lives. Food is at the bottom of Maslow's pyramid of needs. It is a basic need, but much more. We celebrate victories and holidays with food. We console ourselves with food after funerals. We use food to celebrate religious ceremonies. Food is an integral part of the human social fabric. Food defines us as peoples and as cultures. We eat to console ourselves, often when we are bored or upset. There is no food to compare with what our own Mother's served us when growing up. We can remember the flavor, texture and aroma of food for the rest of our lives and often are nostalgic for foods we ate when young or on a special occasion. We call foods that are warm or pleasurable 'comfort foods'. Warm stews for dinner on a cold winter night or a refreshingly cold borsht on a hot summer day are good examples.

What is the sense of denying ourselves the comfort of foods that are so much a part of our lives? I jokingly suggest to my friends that a chocolate covered donut (Entenmann's® of course!) is health food. Yes, it is high in fat and sugar. But eating it is an experience that can make us happy, if we can just relax and enjoy it. The texture and flavor are wonderful. And since being happy makes us healthy, it is therefore a health food! I am, of course saying this with some levity, but eating a chocolate covered donut is pleasurable. If we adjust our diet for the fat and sugar we ingested, we can suffer no long or short term negative consequences. Eating such a donut every day of our lives might be excessive, but once a week certainly won't kill us, especially if we balance our overall diet to appropriately compensate. There are no good or bad foods, only bad diets. If we balance our diets, we can even eat a chocolate covered donut without harm. I don't want to be lying on my deathbed bemoaning the fact that I unnecessarily denied myself the joy of eating a few donuts in my lifetime! Let's learn how to balance our diets, so we can eat the foods we love, even if some food guru says that they are unhealthy.

Designing a Recipe

It is useful, when selecting the ingredients to include in a recipe, to consider that each ingredient plays a different role to produce the desired nutrition, flavor, aroma and texture. There are three basic categories of ingredients: those that are characterizing, those that are complementary and those that contribute. This is true just as true for nutrition as for flavor, texture and aroma.

Characterizing ingredients are the main players that dominate the recipe in nutrition, flavor, aroma or texture, or possibly all four. These are the ingredients that define the recipe. We want them to be obvious and define the character of the recipe. For example: when we eat a steak, we want to taste, smell and feel the texture of the steak. Adding another ingredient to a steak that is stronger in flavor or aroma, would detract from the steak. We can add complementary or contributing ingredients like pepper, salt, mushrooms, blue cheese, onions or even a savory steak sauce, but not another dominant ingredient like ketchup!

Complementary ingredients are side players that are strong enough to be detected in flavor, aroma or texture, but complement the characterizing ingredient. Adding ripe, sliced pears or even pine nuts to a salad, complement the flavor and texture of the leafy green we are using, especially if the leafy part of the salad is something bitter like endive, radicchio or arugula. The sweetness of the pear and the nuttiness of the pine nuts complement the bitter flavor of the endive. These flavors are obvious and add to the complexity of the salad in a pleasant manner without detracting from the flavor of the characterizing ingredient. Complementary ingredients are excellent for boosting the antioxidant and fiber content of a recipe. Some versatile ingredients that can help you to do this effectively include: cinnamon, cocoa powder, ginger root fresh or powder, clove powder, turmeric, chia seeds, pine nuts, pistachio nuts, and balsamic vinegar.

Contributing ingredients are background players that enhance but are not noticeable in flavor, aroma or texture. They do not stick out above the other ingredients, but rather add additional background notes. These can be strongly flavored ingredients that are used at a low enough level so as not to be obvious, but only enhance. For example: dried ginger powder is a great enhancer that contributes a bright, spicy note to a salad or soup. When used at a low level the flavor of ginger itself is not characterizing or obvious, but still contributes flavor and beneficial antioxidants. Vanilla is another great example of a contributing flavor that we use liberally in baking, beverages and desserts, because it is a wonderful enhancing flavor. At high, characterizing levels, vanilla becomes bitter and chemical tasting. Even in vanilla ice cream, the vanilla note is at best complementing the sweet dairy notes. The quintessential example of a recipe with contributing notes is Coca Cola. The ingredients in Coca Cola of course are a top secret, but it is well known that they include cinnamon, coca bean and vanilla among others. These ingredients are difficult to define in the flavor of Coke, because they are perfectly balanced and blended so that no single note sticks out to be characterizing. All the flavors present in Coke are contributing so that we cannot detect the individual ingredients, but all contribute to creating the iconic flavor of Coke. The point is to learn how to add contributing ingredients to your recipes to enhance nutrition, flavor, texture and aroma.

It is important to use good ingredients. Good does not mean expensive, it means in good condition as appropriate to what we are trying to achieve. An example is choosing the right degree of ripeness in a pear. If we are using it in a pie, we want the pear to be firm and crispy, so that it stands up to the baking. If we are using pears in a salad, we probably want a more ripe and soft pear where the sweet flavor and soft texture of the pear blend in nicely with the salad. Or maybe, we want a firm, crispy pear that we can slice very thin so that it blends in with the lettuce better. The condition of the ingredient is important to consider. Using, limp, rubbery broccoli can never be good and no amount of kitchen wizardry will improve it. We can ruin a good ingredient with improper technique, but rarely, can good technique recover a poor ingredient. Consider the condition of the ingredient and what effects of flavor, texture and aroma we are trying to achieve with it.

Don't be afraid to experiment. Sometimes the pears are too firm or we don't have all the ingredients that we need, but have some others that may substitute. Adjust as appropriate and aim for a good final result in spite of the challenges. Who knows, we might like it better!

What does all this have to do with good nutrition and diet? Our goal is to change the way we eat in order to change our lives. Living a longer, healthier, vibrant life will require that we get the diet piece right, not only because of the nutrients it delivers but also because of the enjoyment we get from eating. In order to be sustainable as a set of changes that we make and keep for the rest of our lives, the changes need to fit our lifestyle and be enjoyable. We have learned over and over again, that people will stay on an inconvenient or unenjoyable diet for a limited period of time and then go back to what they know best. Our goal is to change what we know and make it our new normal. We will still deviate occasionally, but when we come back, this new and improved diet is what we will come back to. We will incorporate new ingredients into our existing diet and add some new meals. The result will be a change we can live with and enjoy. It will consistently deliver moderate levels of carbs, protein and fat; with high fiber and antioxidants. It will make us look and feel better. It will make us want to live longer, because we are feeling better. It will prevent the diseases of the Metabolic Syndrome. We don't want to go there. Remember, we don't want care, we want cure. Now that is a vision!

Constructing a Meal

We should think about each meal, the components in it and how each contributes to the total nutrition of the meal. A meal is constructed from individual foods that we select for nutrition, flavor and pure enjoyment. Eating can be fun, satisfying and nutritional all at the same time. The idea is to combine foods that allow us to achieve a nutritional balance of calories, fats, protein, carbs, sugar, fiber, ORAC, omega-3's, etc. It's really not rocket science, or even very complicated. If we learn how to eat a balanced diet, composed of many different foods, and add some new, functional ingredients to our potpourri, we can get there!

First let's discuss a little background information on the approach we will take. Recent topics of discussion in nutrition circles include the concepts of nutrient density and satiety. The suggestion is to consume highly nutrient dense foods. What this means is to select foods that are high in good nutrients like protein, healthy fats, moderate in carbs and low in sugar. Satiety is the feeling of fullness we get from eating a food. Foods vary in the degree to which they make our bellies feel full. If we eat foods that are high in satiety, the idea is that we will eat less. Sometimes that doesn't work so well, enabling overeating. On the other hand, eating low nutrient density foods will allow us to eat more, and feel satisfied while keeping caloric intake low. Satiety and nutrient density are both interesting technical concepts, but may be difficult to implement in our daily dietary choice, so let's consider a simpler approach.

It takes about 500 to 600 grams of food to make our bellies feel satisfied. Notice that I didn't say stuffed! We don't want to overeat. Too much of a good thing is not a good thing. We want to select foods that provide the nutrients our bodies need in the right balance, without too many calories. The table below shows reasonable target values for the grams of food, calories, grams of carbs, grams of protein and grams of fat in a meal, depending on whether we are eating two or three meals a day.

Assuming we will eat 2 meals a day, good targets to aim for in a meal are:

2 Meals/Day	Grams	Calories	Carbs Grams	Protein Grams	Fat Grams
Lunch	500	1000	150	50	22
Dinner	750	1500	225	75	33
Total	1250	2500	375	125	55

If we are eating 3 meals a day, the totals stay the same, just distributed differently. This is why it's best to get down to eating 2 meals a day. When we eat three meals, it will be difficult to reduce breakfast and lunch enough to avoid overeating.

3 Meals/Day	Grams	Calories	Carbs Grams	Protein Grams	Fat Grams
Breakfast	150	300	45	15	7
Lunch	350	700	105	35	15
Dinner	750	1500	225	75	33
Total	1250	2500	375	125	55

The following table compares two meal choices. One is a McDonalds® meal and the other is our Special Salad (the recipe is in Appendix 1).

	Weight (grams)	Calories	Total Fat (grams)	Saturated Fat (grams)	Total Carbs (grams)	Omega-3 (grams)	Sugar (grams)	Fiber (grams)	ORAC (umol TE)	Protein (grams)	Cholesterol (mg)
McDonalds Double Quarter Pounder w/Cheese, Medium Fries and Medium Coke	488	1290	58	22	145	Low	68	7	? Low	51	165
Special Salad	508	681	52	6	53	3	18	23	12,382	7	0

This simple table has only two meals in it for easy comparison – a McDonalds® meal comprised of a Double Quarter Pounder® with cheese, medium fries and a medium Coke®, compared to our special salad. Let's consider these two alternative meals as options for lunch or dinner. Both will fill you up with about 500 grams of food. But that's where the similarities end! The calories of the special salad are half, total fat is about the same, but the quality of the fat is totally different, saturated fat is reduced by over 4X, carbs are reduced by 3X, the salad provides over half of your required omega-3, fiber is over triple, ORAC is off the charts and cholesterol is zero for the salad. Change the Coke® for a Diet Coke® or water and the sugar and carbs in the McDonalds® meal drop by 45 grams along with 180 calories. The only way the McDonalds® meal beats our special salad is in protein – providing over 7 times the protein. But we can design breakfast and lunch to provide plenty of protein.

This comparison points out the differences between an indulgent McDonalds® meal and a mixed salad. And just for the record, I occasionally eat at McDonalds®, and the Double Quarter Pounder® is my favorite! As long as we balance the calories and fat over the next few days, we can eat a McDonalds® meal without any harm. When I come home after a few weeks in a country in Asia that I won't mention at the risk of offending someone, the first thing I do when I get off the plane is head to a McDonalds® for this meal. It recalibrates me. When you need a McDonalds® hit, go for it, and as a steady diet, go with the special salad!

The next step is to design other meal choices that meet our nutritional needs and are fun and fit our lifestyle. The goal is to minimize carb intake in the morning to extend our nighttime fast until lunch, or even better to eat two meals a day and skip breakfast. At lunch and dinner, we need to increase the carbs to support our metabolic needs. If we are mostly sedentary that day, keep the carbs at around 350 grams total for lunch and dinner. If you are active physically, then feel free to increase carbs as needed. It's hard to estimate the amount of carbs that each person needs, since there are so many factors involved. This is why it's important that we know our own body. The most effective way for us to assess if we are on balance with carb intake is to look at our body. Are we carrying around excess baggage in belly or leg fat? If yes, then reduce carb intake, and use a scale to assess progress. If not, then maintain what you are doing. If we are too skinny and don't have enough body fat, then increase carb intake. Carbs are the gas pedal that we use to control speed.

Transforming Ordinary into Extraordinary!

The goal is to take ordinary meals and transform them into extraordinary meals that meet our nutritional, cultural and lifestyle needs. We want to learn how to substitute ingredients as needed to cope with availability, economics, personal preference or just for the sake of variety. Have some fun with it!

Let's start with a breakfast meal – oat bran. Oat bran is a good choice as it is high in beta glucan fiber, moderate in carbs, very low in sugar, it's inexpensive, widely available, it tastes good and can be modified to our taste. I prefer a coarsely milled oat bran cereal, as I like the texture better and it cooks up with less lumps than the finely milled varieties.

How can we transform an oat bran breakfast from ordinary to extraordinary?

- First, let's start with our oat bran cereal – 40 grams (3 tablespoons dry)
- Add 13 grams (1 tablespoon) of Chia seeds. This adds omega-3 fat, increases the fiber even more, adds antioxidants and adds an interesting texture of the seeds.
- For good antioxidants let's add 7.4 grams (1 tablespoon) cocoa powder, and 6 grams (1 teaspoon) of ground cinnamon. If you are really adventurous, a gram (1/3 teaspoon) of ginger powder and a dash of ground cloves will spice it up. These add flavor too. The cloves are strongly flavored and it may take some getting used to, but after eating it a few times, you will like it better. The antioxidant content of cloves is very high, even higher than cinnamon or ginger. Cinnamon is amazingly versatile. You can add a small amount to a dish like this and it is noticeable but not overpowering, and adds a very pleasant, spicy and floral note. Ginger is also amazing as it incorporates well into a dish like this. You will not even notice that it is there. The only evidence of its presence is the slightly hot (picante) note and a brightness of flavor that is unique to ginger and very pleasant. Cocoa powder is mild in flavor and easy to incorporate into many different recipes.

- Good oils are still missing in this dish. Except for the Chia seeds, everything we have added so far is low in fat of any kind. So, let's add 45 grams (3 tablespoons of walnut oil). Walnut oil has a pleasant nutty flavor and is a healthy oil with a low melting point.

- Add 200 grams of water (7 ounces) and stir. I like to microwave it in 45 second increments until it is rising like a cake, stirring in between each. If you don't like microwave ovens, then boil the water first and add it to the oat bran and chia seeds.

- Lastly, I like to add a little milk or even half and half cream to help cool it off a bit and to improve the flavor and texture. I typically add 45 grams (3 tablespoons). The amount of saturated fat this adds is not worth mentioning. This is optional.

- See Appendix 4 for the full recipe, and nutritional values.

That's it! Simple enough and we have transformed this meal by adding a significant amount of antioxidants, good oils, increased the fiber, made the texture more interesting and gave it some interesting flavor. That is one way to transform an ordinary meal into an extraordinary one! Notice that we didn't add any kind of sugar. We could add a little sugar, but with some taste-bud training, we can skip the sugar, especially by adding spices. The benefit is we can keep the sugar content of this meal very low and since it is typically a breakfast meal, we can keep our blood glucose level low and allow our bodies to remain in fat metabolism until lunch. Since we haven't eaten anything since dinner last night, this allows us to extend the period of fat metabolism from eight hour to at least twelve hours. And since we are active in the morning, our bodies will need calories and we want those to be fat calories taken from the fat stores in our body. It's time to take some of that fat we deposited in the past out of the bank. All good!

Designing a Diet

Here is a list of a few of the nutritional factors that we need to be aware of when designing a meal or a diet:

- How many grams the meal delivers. Grams matter because this determines how satisfied we will feel after eating. This is why eating a bowl of soup, as is customary in European cuisine, is a great strategy to partially fill the belly with a great tasting soup that is mostly water and contains very few calories. We don't want to starve or be hungry all the time. On the other hand, we need to get accustomed to eating less and not eating until we are full. Remember, overeating is one of the main causes of the Metabolic Syndrome and diabetes.

- How many meals a day we plan to eat. If we can get down to two meals a day, it makes it easier to plan satisfying meals. Avoiding snacking in between meals helps too, as this can add significant calories that we are unlikely to compensate for when we eat the meals. Drinking sugar-free liquids any time helps avoid snacking.

- How many calories the meal or diet delivers. Calories matter! For a sedentary lifestyle, depending on body size (not fat), aim for 2,000 to 2,500 calories total per day. If you are more active, increase the carbs, keeping protein and fat the same. Be careful not to overestimate how many calories you are burning during exercise and work. The human body is remarkably efficient. The best gauge of your need for more carbs is to watch the scale. If you are losing weight and don't want to, then increase carbs. If you are losing weight and need to, don't increase the carbs! Water contains no calories, so drinking more water or sugar-free liquids is an easy way to increase intake without adding calories. There is conflicting evidence on whether artificially sweetened beverages cause an impact on blood glucose – small amounts are unlikely to cause any harm.[33]

- How much protein the meal provides (protein quality is important too, but beyond the scope of this book to consider). Typically, we aim for twenty percent of calories from protein. Protein contains about 4 calories per gram, so a good daily target is 100 to 125 grams of protein each day.

- How much fat, saturated fat, monounsaturated fat, polyunsaturated fat, omega-3 fatty acids, omega-6 fatty acids and cholesterol the meal or diet delivers. Typically, we aim for twenty to forty percent of calories from fats and oils. These contain about 9 calories per gram, so a good daily target is 55 to 100 grams of fats and oils per day.

- How much carbohydrates, sugar and dietary fiber the meal or diet delivers. Typically, aim for forty to sixty percent of calories from carbs. Keep sugar as low as possible. Carbs contain about 4 calories per gram, so a good daily target is 250 to 375 grams of total carbs per day.

- How much vitamins (folate, niacin, pyridoxine (B6), pantothenic acid, riboflavin, Vitamin A, Vitamin C, Vitamin D, Vitamin E and Vitamin K) the meal or diet delivers.

- How much minerals (calcium, sodium, potassium, phosphorus, copper, iron, magnesium, manganese, selenium and zinc) the meal or diet delivers.

- How much antioxidants the meal or diet provides. ORAC is the measure of the quantity of antioxidants in a food. Recommendations on how much antioxidants to consume vary greatly. 5000 um TE/day is a good minimum, but I have seen recommendations up to 5 times that. The science is lacking to establish a good target, but there is some consensus that 25,000 Units per day is good. There is some evidence that too much antioxidants can cause harm as well.[34]

The trick is to find foods that complement each other to provide the necessary nutrients in a reasonable balance while managing caloric intake. Learning how to do this with foods that we can afford, that are available where we shop, that we like to eat and that allow us to mix it up for variety so we're not eating the same foods every day is a real challenge! This is why we must be passionate and be willing to invest the time to become somewhat of an expert on what we eat.

Let's start by looking at some real foods and break down their nutritional content. I've selected some common foods from each category for simplicity. From this we can get an idea of how to build a diet. There is a lot of help available on Apps and websites, including the outstanding USDA Nutrition Database, that is comprehensive and free.

USDA Handbook No. 8 and SR-21 Nutrition Values for Foods

Shrt Desc http://nutritiondata.self.com	Grams of Food per 100 Calories	Percent Water	Calories Per 100 grams of Food	Grams Protein per 100 Grams of Food	Grams Fat per 100 Grams of Food	Grams Carbs per 100 Grams of Food	Grams sugar per 100 Grams of Food	Grams fiber per 100 Grams of Food	ORAC umTE/100 gms
ASPARAGUS,RAW	500	93.22	20	2.2	0.12	3.88	0	2.1	3017
COLLARDS,CKD,BLD,DRND,WO/SALT	385	91.8	26	2.1	0.4	4.9	0.4	2.8	1200
KALE,RAW	357	91.2	28	1.9	0.4	5.63	1.3	2	1770
ARUGULA,RAW	286	90.35	35	0.64	0.13	8.24	2.1	2.9	1900
BROCCOLI,RAW	286	89.25	35	2.38	0.41	7.18	1.7	3.3	1590
CARROTS,RAW	286	90.17	35	0.76	0.18	8.22	1.4	3	1215
OAT BRAN,COOKED	250	84	40	3.21	0.86	11.44	1.7	2.6	2183
APPLES,RAW,WITH SKIN	192	85.56	52	0.26	0.17	13.81	16	2.4	3000
CORN,SWT,YEL,RAW	116	76	86	3.2	1.2	19	3.2	2.7	728
BANANAS,RAW	112	74.91	89	1.09	0.33	22.84	12.2	2.6	879
FISH, SALMON,ATLANTIC,WILD,RAW	85	72	117	18.28	4.32	0	0	0	30
EGG,WHL,RAW,FRSH	70	76.15	143	12.56	9.51	0.72	0.8	0	20
AVOCADOS,RAW,ALL COMM VAR	63	73.23	160	2	14.66	8.53	0.7	6.7	1933
FISH, SALMON,ATLANTIC,FARMED,RAW	49	64.75	206	22.1	12.35	0	0	0	30
BEEF, COMP OF RTL CUTS,LN&FAT,1/8"FAT,CHOIC,CKD	45	63.03	223	18.87	15.75	0	0	0	795
WHOLE WHEAT BREAD, COMMERCIAL	40	38	247	13	3.3	41.3	5.6	6.8	1421
CHEESE, SWISS	26	37.12	380	26.93	27.8	5.38	1.3	0	697
NUTS, PISTACHIO NUTS,DRY RSTD,W/SALT	22	4.5	446	18.55	19.4	53.75	0	18.4	7675
COOKIES, CHOCOLATE CHIP, MADE W BUTTER	18	3	548	6.45	32.3	61.3	35.5	3.2	8750
PEANUTS,ALL TYPES,DRY-ROASTED,W/SALT	18	6.39	570	26.15	49.6	15.82	4.2	9.5	3166
NUTS, WALNUTS,BLACK,DRIED	15	4.07	654	15.23	65.21	13.71	1.1	6.7	13541
PECANS	14	1.12	710	9.5	74.27	13.55	4	9.4	17940
BUTTER, WITH SALT	14	15.87	717	0.85	81.11	0.06	0.1	0	730

Column 2 – Grams of Food per 100 Calories

I've sorted these foods by the Caloric content, with the lowest first and increasing from there. The first column shows how many grams of the food it takes to contain 100 calories.

- The first on the food on the list is asparagus with 500 grams required to deliver 100 calories. That is a lot of asparagus! Why is it so low in calories? First notice that it is 93 percent water. It is also very low in fat (0.12%), has no measurable sugar, has 2.1% fiber and a respectable ORAC value of 3017.
- Most veggies are low in calories, and here I have included arugula, kale, broccoli and carrots, which are high in water content (over 90%), are low in fat (less than 0.4%), low in sugar (less than 2%), moderate in fiber (2-3%) and good sources of antioxidants (1200-3000 ORAC). Carrots get a bad rap for containing sugar. This is nonsense, as carrots have no more sugar than any other vegetable, and the little sugar they contain is well worth it considering the benefits of low calories, good fiber, good antioxidants, Vitamin A (16,705 IU/100 gm), potassium (320 mg/100 gm), not to mention great flavor, texture and crunch. Foods that are high in water content naturally contain less calories and the bulk helps to fill up our bellies, making us feel satisfied sooner. All good things.
- Next we get to grains, fruits, fish, meats and whole wheat bread. These foods are moderate in caloric content, due to the high-water content, (60-90%) as eaten. We don't eat grains raw, thank God! When grains like oat bran are cooked, they absorb a lot of water that adds bulk and keeps calories low. Grains and the foods made from them, like whole wheat bread, are great sources of complex carbs, fiber

and protein, with moderate caloric content, good ORAC values and low in sugar.

- The high caloric value foods include cheese, nuts, cookies and finally butter. Dried cheeses are higher in calories because the moisture content is low. Unaged cheeses like cottage cheese or mozzarella are higher in water content and lower in calories. Nuts are low in water content and high in fat, giving them high caloric values. And butter is mostly fat (80%), making it high in calories. But that doesn't make it bad! It only means that we should consume it in moderation, with awareness of the calories it brings. But it also brings great flavor, texture, moderates sugar absorption and provides butyric acid, that is good for our brains![28]

Please note that these are all 'Good' foods! By being aware of the tradeoffs of water content, calories, and beneficial nutrients, we can construct a balanced and nutritious diet that contains all of these foods and many others.

Column 5 – Grams of Protein per 100 Grams of Food

This column is not sorted, so protein levels vary by food. A few important points to notice:

- Veggies and fruits are low in protein (0.26-2.38%)
- Grains are moderate in protein content (3.21%)
- Eggs are moderately high in protein content (12%)
- Meats and fish are high in protein (18-22%)
- Nuts and whole wheat bread are high in protein (10-26%)
- Cheese (dried) is very high in protein (26.83%)

We need to include these foods in our diet to get the protein we need.

Column 6 – Grams of Fat per 100 Grams of Food

The fat content of foods vary widely from:

- Very low in veggies and fruits (0.12-0.41%), with the exception of avocados at 14.66%
- Moderate in whole wheat bread, eggs, meat and fish (3.3-15%)
- High in dried cheese (27%)
- Very high in nuts (50-74%), with the exception of pistachio nuts at 19.4%.
- Butter, fats and oils are almost 100% fat.

Don't be afraid of fat. All the hype about saturated fats being bad for us has finally been proven wrong, as long as our diet also contains adequate amounts of the low melting point oils that we get from nuts and fish. **Fat doesn't cause heart disease. Fat doesn't cause heart disease.** I said it twice, and put it in bold type, because the opposite has been drummed into our heads for the past 30 years. We have been given bad advice. Very bad, because if we eat less fat, then we must eat more carbs (usually sugar) and protein. The protein is not an issue, but the higher carbs and sugar certainly are. And fat helps reduce the blood glucose spike caused by eating high carb foods. I didn't say high sugar for a reason. Fat is good! Fat will help us avoid diabetes. And can I say it again? **Fat doesn't cause heart disease!** Even trans fats are no longer a risk, as the partial hydrogenation process that produced them has been banned, and the naturally occurring trans fats in meat and butter aren't a risk. My dear friend Bill Knightly was a fat chemist (he wasn't fat, but what he studied was!). He presciently told me years ago that the issue with fat and heart disease was melting point. Saturated fats have higher melting points than monounsaturated and polyunsaturated fats. Coconut oil melts at 75 to 85 degrees F., butter melts at 80 to 92 degrees F., and Cocoa butter melts at 93 to 98 degrees F. These are all below or close to body temperature, so shouldn't be a problem in the body – and they are not a problem. Some common trans fats have melting points of 150 degrees F, much higher than body temperature, and that was part of the problem. But cholesterol, which our bodies produce at the rate of about 4 grams a day, has a melting point of 250 degrees F – much higher than body temperature. As long as we have sufficient lower melting point fatty acids in our bloodstream to keep cholesterol moving, there is no problem. This is why the advice to reduce fat intake, including even good fats like olive oil, nut oils and fish oil, was so bad. And remember those short chain fatty acids that our intestinal bacteria make when they are happy and fed properly – acetic acid, butyric acid, propionic acid? Those also help prevent cholesterol, and other high melting point fats from causing heart disease. Are you ready to kiss your intestinal bacteria yet?! And besides all that, fat is a required nutrient, so we want fat in our diet for lots of reasons.

Column 7, 8 and 9 – Grams of Carbs, Sugar and Fiber per 100 Grams of Food

The carb value in column 7 is total carbs, which includes the complex carbs, sugar and fiber, as these are all carbs. We need to separate these in order to minimize the sugar in our diet, get a moderate amount of complex carbs and increase fiber as much as possible.

- Meat, fish, eggs, and all animal products have no or very low carbs. This sounds good, but they also have no fiber. In a balanced diet this is not a problem, as we can select other foods to contribute the fiber we need.
- Vegetables are low in carbs (3.9 to 8.2%), very low in sugar (0 to 2.1%) and contain a significant amount of fiber (2 to 3.3%). Even 'evil' carrots, at 8% total carbs, contain only 1.4% sugar and deliver 3% fiber.

- Fermented products like hard cheeses and yogurt will be low in sugar, unless it is being added (read the label) as fermentation digests the sugar.
- Fruits and corn are moderate in carbs at 11.4 to 22.8%, have 12.2 to 16% sugar and 2.4 to 2.6% fiber.
- Nuts are moderate in carbs, low in sugar and high in fiber.
- Baked goods are high in carbs (41.3 to 61.3%), mostly complex carbs that take time to digest and absorb. Whole wheat bread is low in sugar at 5.6% and high in fiber at 6.8%. Most of the carbs are complex carbs such as starch that take time to digest, slowing the release of glucose. No surprise, ordinary chocolate chip cookies are high in sugar (35.5%). Not mine – by the way! More about that later.

Column 10 – ORAC per 100 Grams of Food

ORAC stands for the Oxidation Radical Absorbance Capacity and is reported in µmole TE per 100 grams. This is a measure of the oxidative capacity of the food. µmole means micro moles, and TE stands for Trolox Equivalent, which is a type of vitamin E, used as a standard in the analysis. Suffice it to say that antioxidants are a good thing in the diet, preventing chronic inflammation of tissues and damage to the body from free radicals, which are highly reactive chemicals formed by contact with oxygen. Believe it or not, oxygen is actually a poison to life. Early life was strictly anaerobic, meaning free from oxygen. Life had to find a way to deal with oxygen, when it started building up in the early atmosphere, and the solution was to harness it to enhance energy production in the cell, while controlling it with antioxidants to prevent harm.[35] Good for us that plants produce a lot of antioxidants to protect themselves and us from the negative effects of oxygen.

- Meat, fish, eggs and most animal products are low in antioxidants with ORAC values ranging from 20 in eggs to 795 in beef and butter.
- Vegetables contain moderate amounts of antioxidants (1200 to 3017 ORAC). This includes peanuts, which of course are actually a legume. Grains are also moderate and whole wheat bread contains 1421 ORAC.
- The real stars of antioxidants are the nuts and dark colored fruits such as blueberries and raspberries. Even chocolate chip cookies deliver 8750 ORAC due to the cocoa in the chocolate chips. Cocoa, cinnamon, turmeric, ginger and cloves are the most potent antioxidant foods. Nuts are particularly great in the diet, as they are high in ORAC, high in low melting point fats, high in fiber and very low in sugar. All good.

Most of us think that a good meal, and therefore diet, is composed of a piece of meat or fish in the center of the plate, some carbs like potatoes, rice or pasta, and then to garnish the plate with a vegetable like corn or peas. This is backwards thinking. Instead, we should place the vegetables at the center of the plate, but not corn or peas please, as these are too high in carbs. Start with a healthy portion of vegetables that are moderate in carbs, low in calories and sugar and high in fiber and antioxidants, such as asparagus, broccoli, broccoli rabe, brussels sprouts, kale, cabbage, or collards. Then add a carb, but choose one that is high in fiber and low in sugar, such as whole wheat bread served with butter, olive oil or just balsamic vinegar for dipping. Finally, add a small piece of meat or fish for protein.

When I was growing up, we were told, like in the Pink Floyd song "Another Brick in the Wall", that we had to eat the meat. For us today, this is also backwards thinking. There is nothing wrong with eating meat, from a nutritional perspective, ethics and environmental sustainability notwithstanding. However; the point is that we would get more fiber and antioxidants, if we ate less meat and more veggies. We would also do better to start the meal with soup and vegetables. This approach will allow us to eat a satisfying meal, while keeping calories low, sugar low, protein moderate, carbs moderate, fiber high, and antioxidants high. Serving a bowl of broth soup (not a cream-based soup or bisque) before the meal is even better. Heat bone broth or chicken stock with some leafy green vegetables like arugula, endive or escarole. It couldn't be much easier and it tastes great.

Getting Fiber into Our Diet

If we are going to make a real change in the health of our intestinal microbiome, we need to increase our daily fiber intake up to over fifty grams. Most people on a western diet are getting around eleven grams per day. We literally don't know how to go from eleven to fifty. We need to learn how to get that much fiber and make the changes in our daily diet to put it there and keep it there, every day, for the rest of our lives. Let's consider the options. I'm going to focus on foods and recipes that deliver at least ten grams of fiber per serving or meal. We must do this!

- First we can eat green vegetables that are high in fiber. The Special Salad recipe in Appendix 1 delivers 19 grams of fiber. Not so bad for one meal, already 40% of our goal. We can eat asparagus, broccoli, broccoli rabe, brussels sprouts, kale, Swiss chard, collards – all contain 2-3 grams of fiber per 100 grams serving. That is part of the problem. To get ten grams of fiber, we have to eat a pound of green vegetables. That's too much. We need to do better.
- We can eat oat bran cereal. A cup of cooked oat bran delivers about 3 grams of fiber. It is mostly beta glucan, which is one of the best fibers we can eat, because it does more than just feed our microbiome. This is good, but not going to get us

to 50 grams. We can boost the fiber by adding cinnamon powder, cocoa powder and chia seeds. Cinnamon is about 50% fiber, cocoa powder and chia seeds are about 33% fiber. A tablespoon of cocoa powder weighs about 7.4 grams and delivers 2.4 grams of fiber. A teaspoon of cinnamon powder weights about 6 grams and delivers 3 grams of fiber. A tablespoon of chia seeds weigh about 13 grams and delivers 4 grams of fiber. By adding a tablespoon of cocoa powder, a tablespoon of chia seeds and a teaspoon of cinnamon powder to our three tablespoons of dry oat bran cereal in a cup of water, will not only make it taste a lot better but increase the fiber per serving from three grams up to 12.4 grams. We are now in the ballpark!

- There are now available several very good high fiber cereals that deliver up to 16 grams of fiber per serving. This is a good addition to our diet, as it gets us almost a third of the way towards our goal of 50 grams per day. And best of all they taste good and can fit our lifestyle without any sacrifices. One of them is called "Poop Like a Champion ™" – no need to say any more than that!

- We can eat nuts. Most nuts have about 10% fiber, so to get 10 grams of fiber we need to eat 100 grams. That is possible, but delivers a lot of calories (600 to 700). Pistachios are 18% fiber, so we only need to eat 55 grams and that will have 245 calories. Now we're in the ballpark. 55 grams of shelled pistachio nuts are about 1/3 cup by volume or 4 good handfuls.

- Psyllium husk fiber is convenient, as it is almost pure fiber, has no flavor and is easy on the digestive system. It comes in two forms – whole flake and powder. Nutritionally they are the same, but the powder form absorbs water voraciously and quickly, forming a strong gel. The whole flake form will also absorb a lot of water, but it does so more slowly, making it possible to mix it into a cup of water and drink it down before it turns into a gel. Twelve grams of whole flake or powdered psyllium husk will deliver 10 grams of fiber. I fast until 11 AM, with only coffee before that, have a psyllium shake at 11 AM and eat pistachio nuts or a few pieces of bitter unsweetened chocolate at 4 PM. This gives me lots of fiber, no sugar, very few calories and I'm not hungry until dinner time, enabling me to achieve a 22-hour fast once a week. Watch your blood glucose level – mine doesn't budge after the psyllium shake. See Appendix 6 for an improved recipe.

- Chocolate is a great food to incorporate as an ingredient and for snacking in order to increase fiber and antioxidants. Slowly train your taste buds to accept chocolate with higher and higher levels of cocoa and therefore, more fiber and less sugar. The 60% and 85% cocoa chocolates contain about ten % fiber, and the bitter or unsweetened chocolate contains about sixteen % fiber.

- It is important that we have access to foods we like to eat and also deliver fiber, and that is why I have developed a chocolate cookie recipe that delivers ten grams of fiber per 50-gram cookie with only five grams of sugar. It is low in sugar and tastes great. I eat one for dessert after dinner when I feel the need. The recipe contains polydextrose, which is water soluble and has no flavor. It is one of the easiest fibers to digest, meaning it will not likely cause any intestinal distress as you add it to your diet. Polydextrose powder is available online. The first time you eat these cookies, if your intestines are not up to par, you may experience some flatulence, but that will go away after a few days. I personally had no problem. This is how we can create foods that we like to eat and deliver the fiber we need. One of these cookies will provide 10 grams of fiber – that is probably double what you eat now in a whole day. This is a game changer. And I would rather eat a great tasting cookie than drink a slimy psyllium goo. But that's just me! You can bake these cookies yourself, using the recipe in Appendix 3, or they are available from The

Biome Bakery ™ at www.biomebaking.com. These cookies have been formulated on purpose to moderate the absorption of sugar and to have a minimal impact on blood glucose.

- Another easy food to incorporate into our everyday diet and lifestyle is a bagel. For that purpose, I have also developed a bagel made with whole wheat flour, that delivers 14 grams of total fiber, one gram as beta glucan, 25 mg of lutein antioxidant, 10 grams of flaxseed meal to provide essential fatty acids (linoleic and linolenic), while having less than one gram of sugar. Most of the fiber is resistant wheat starch which is easy on the digestive system. It also contains activated charcoal powder, which has been shown to protect the intestinal bacteria by absorbing toxic materials that are present in food. I think they are great! These are also available from The Biome Bakery ™ at www.biomebaking.com.

- Experiment and learn how to incorporate fiber into your own recipes. The easiest ingredients to do this are probably already in your pantry! The point is that a little extra fiber here and there adds up to real numbers. This can be fun, taste great and make you a better cook. Here are some examples:

  o Cocoa powder: 33% fiber and very high in ORAC – can be sprinkled on or added to almost any recipe and it tastes great. A tablespoon adds 2.4 grams of fiber. Unsweetened chocolate is also great for fiber at sixteen %. A 20-gram piece of unsweetened chocolate gives you over 3 grams of fiber and almost no sugar. A great snack. And once you get used to eating it without sugar, you will cringe at how sweet regular chocolate is.

  o Cinnamon powder: 50% fiber and very high in ORAC – can be sprinkled on or added to almost any recipe and it tastes great. A teaspoon adds 3 grams of fiber. Limit total daily consumption to

2 teaspoons per day. I find cinnamon powder to irritate my stomach, so I use cocoa instead.

o Sprinkle a few nuts on almost anything – salads, veggies, even pasta! Nuts are around 10% fiber so 20 grams of nuts, which is a handful, will add 2 grams of fiber. Walnuts, pine nuts, pecans, almonds, cashews, etc. are all good. Pistachio nuts are best due to having lower fat and higher fiber content than the other nuts.

o Chia seeds: 33% fiber and high in omega-3 fatty acids. Chia seeds can be sprinkled on almost any recipe – salads, veggies, mashed potatoes, etc. A tablespoon adds 4 grams of fiber. Did you know that you can make an added-sugar free jam by using fresh fruit and chia seeds? There is still plenty of sugar in the fruit – so be careful. But, there is no additional sugar needed to make a jam, when using chia seeds. That is a significant reduction in sugar. Just add a tablespoon of chia seeds to a cupful of fruit, puree in a blender and cook until thick. When it cools, it will gel very nicely.

o Psyllium husk whole flakes: almost 100% fiber, have no real flavor and can be sprinkled onto almost anything. The flakes will absorb a lot of water if it is available. On a salad, that is not a problem. When you are making lasagna (see Appendix 5 for a kale lasagna) you can sprinkle a bit of psyllium husk whole flakes as you create the layers. It has the added benefit of absorbing water as it cooks, so if you ever made lasagna that was watery – with this technique it will not be watery! Anything that you normally add bread crumbs to can benefit from psyllium husk whole flakes or chia seeds as these will absorb water just like the bread crumbs. For example: meatloaf, meatballs, and crab cakes.

To summarize how to get over 50 grams of fiber into your diet:

Every day:

- 100 grams of a green leafy vegetable with your dinner: 3 grams of fiber
- One chocolate chip cookie (50 grams) Special High Fiber, Low Sugar recipe in Appendix 3: 10 grams of fiber, with 210 calories, 6 grams of protein, 14 grams of fat, 25 grams of carbs, 5 grams of sugar and 5,700 ORAC units. These are available from The Biome Bakery ™ at <u>www.biomebaking.com</u>.
- 100 grams of Biome Bakery ™ All-In Biome Balance ™ Bagel: 14 grams of fiber and 6 grams of protein, 6 grams of fat, with only 170 calories, 36 grams of carbs, and less than 0.5 grams of sugar. These are also available from The Biome Bakery ™ at <u>www.biomebaking.com</u>.
- Psyllium husk whole flake or psyllium husk powder shake: 10 grams of fiber

Then pick one of these every day:

- A large salad like the Special Salad in Appendix 1: 19 grams of fiber
- Oat bran cereal with cocoa powder, chia seeds and cinnamon powder: 12.4 grams of fiber
- 50 grams of pistachio nuts: 10 grams of fiber
- A serving of a high fiber cereal: 16 grams of fiber

I eat one of the bagels every day, either with lunch or dinner, with butter, cream cheese, mayonnaise or if I want to eliminate the fat, dip it in balsamic vinegar. This alone give me 14 grams of fiber, so in combination with the psyllium shake in the morning, veggies, and a high fiber cookie for dessert after dinner, I'm at 37 grams of fiber. By adding oat bran cereal, the Special Salad or pistachio nuts, I can break the 50-gram barrier. By adding a few grams of cocoa, ginger or cinnamon here and there as we prepare meals will add up too. Sometimes I cheat and just have a second cookie! Or double up on the psyllium shake. Get creative and design your own recipes with fiber. We can do this! Every day. Just think how happy your intestinal microbiome will be.

Conclusions About Diet

A few critical points to keep in mind as we select what to eat:

- Some foods are better than others, but there are no bad foods, only bad diets. If we manage what we eat and compensate for the occasional indiscretion, we can eat almost anything. Quantity is more important than what we eat. Calories matter.
- Always include low caloric content foods in your diet. Soup and vegetables are great ways to fill up the belly, while delivering beneficial fiber and antioxidants.
- Fruits and grains, including whole wheat bread, are good to have in the diet for fiber, complex carbs, antioxidants and for sheer enjoyment.
- Meats, fish and cheese are good for protein.
- Nuts are great for delivering protein, low melting point oils, antioxidants, and fiber, but are high in calories. A handful is fantastic.
- Select foods that have at least two to three times as much fiber as sugar.
- Spices and seasonings such as cocoa, cinnamon, ginger, turmeric and cloves are great for delivering antioxidants.
- Pistachio nuts and unsweetened chocolate are great for snacking, when you absolutely cannot make it to the next meal, or to replace a meal.

- Cocoa powder, cinnamon powder, chia seeds, nuts and psyllium husk whole flakes can be sprinkled onto almost any recipe with beneficial results in texture, flavor, ORAC and fiber content.
- The magic number for fiber is 50 grams daily. That is probably five times your current intake. Eating more broccoli won't do it! Start off slow and increase your intake until you are consistently, every day above 50 grams. Design you own recipes using high fiber ingredients like polydextrose, psyllium, chia seeds, cocoa, nuts and oat bran. They work! Make these ingredients part of your diet. We are not dieting. We are building a diet that is sustainable and enjoyable for the rest of our lives. Your intestines will be singing, not to mention pooping very happily!

The real beauty of achieving a lifestyle change where we are sustainably and easily consuming a diet high in fiber and antioxidants every day, is that what we eat and when become less and less important. Quantity still matters. Chronic overeating and high sugar consumption are unhealthy and must be avoided. But, you will find your weight, blood glucose and blood pressure automatically going in the right direction. And if we want to overeat once in a while, or eat a donut, we can do it without causing harm. When our body is in balance and in control it is able to safely manage the occasional deviation in diet without harm. This is where we want to be. It requires a few changes:

- High fiber diet containing 50 grams per day from a variety of sources including vegetables, resistant starch in bread, polydextrose (in the cookies), nuts (especially pistachio nuts), oat bran, spices (cocoa, cinnamon, turmeric), and psyllium husk.
- High antioxidant diet containing a target of 25,000 ORAC units per day from a variety of sources. This is not so hard to

do when you consider that our Special Salad alone delivers over 14,000 units! Turmeric and cinnamon have about 1,400 units per gram, so about 5,000 units per teaspoon. Cocoa and dark chocolate deliver about 500 units per gram. Don't get too hung up on ORAC numbers. There is building evidence that the number is not as meaningful as once thought. Meaning, the ORAC value doesn't always correlate to the antioxidant value in the body. Our bodies are very good chemists and change many ingredients into more functional forms. We just need to provide the building blocks in our diet.

- Balance – eat a variety of foods, the broader the better. And when you do overeat or eat something with sugar in it, compensate by adjusting your diet over the next few days to get your overall diet for that time into alignment with your goals. Watch the scale – it doesn't lie!
- Exercise, activity, moving, skipping for joy!
- And enjoying life – attitude, life force.

Timing

Timing when we eat allows the blood glucose system to cycle between glucose and fat metabolism. This is a healthy thing to do in order to increase insulin sensitivity and keep the amount of stored fat in the liver and muscles below the point of causing insulin resistance. We will talk in depth about how to do this in Chapter 8. Basically, there are two modes of metabolism: glucose metabolism and fat metabolism. Our bodies are in one mode or the other. Either we are using glucose to power our bodies or we are using fat. Interestingly, our bodies will not use fat when there is glucose around. What we eat and when, determines which mode we are in.

Eating by the clock is one of the worst things we can do. Of course, we all do it because it is convenient and often socially responsible to eat when everyone else is eating. When we must eat by the clock, try to eat low carbohydrate foods like meat, and bulky foods like salads and veggies. Not carb free, but low to moderate carbs. It is best to eat only when we are hungry and not according to the clock. This allows the mechanisms in our body that control satiety and food intake to work. Hunger is the body telling us that we have depleted blood glucose. The absence of hunger tells us the opposite – blood glucose levels are adequate and there is no need to eat. We don't always need to or want to respond to hunger by eating. We want our bodies to occasionally go into fat metabolism, even if only for a few hours. After a few hours in fat metabolism we will eventually start to feel hungry again. We probably haven't depleted our store of fat (unlikely) but we have accomplished our goal and can celebrate (a little) by eating. And yes – food does taste better when we are hungry!

Breakfast – the Most Important Meal (Not)

I often hear people state that breakfast is the most important meal. Nutritionists and even doctors will say this. It is a myth. An extended overnight and morning fast is the way to get our body into glycogen and fat metabolism, allowing blood glucose and insulin levels to drop to baseline. The worst thing we can do in the morning is have a big glass of juice or a pile of pancakes with syrup!

There are several important benefits to an extended overnight fast. Our blood glucose level will naturally drop as the glucose from the last meal we ate is absorbed and depleted. Soon after the blood glucose level drops, blood insulin level will also drop. This will occur while we are sleeping so we won't feel hungry. If we wake up in the middle of the night, we need to avoid eating anything. Drink some water and then go back to sleep. The low blood insulin level switches the body from glucose metabolism to fat metabolism. This is the way our body was designed to work. Our body will break down some of the fat that we have stored. Yea! This is a good thing.

The second benefit of an extended overnight fast is that it allows us to reset the glucose control system. Blood glucose and insulin levels fall to baseline. And, very importantly, insulin sensitivity improves.[36] The control mechanism works better and the beta cells that produce insulin in the pancreas get to take a beneficial rest.[37]

The third benefit to an extended overnight fast is that it will reduce our intake of calories. As we get older our metabolism slows and for lots of reasons we simply are not as active as we used to be. Watch a 5-year old run around and you will appreciate this. The simple fact of the matter is that we need to reduce our intake of calories or gain weight. It's often not easy or comfortable. Nobody likes starvation diets. Most of us love to eat and even live to eat. Eating is social and cultural and difficult to control. Eliminating one meal a day may give us the ability to eat more freely at lunch and dinner. We can still enjoy eating, maybe even have dessert while being able to achieve and maintain a good body weight.

Some people feel lightheaded or irritable if they don't eat breakfast. This is likely due to insulin resistance – the beginning stage of diabetes. The lightheaded feeling is due to abnormally low levels of blood glucose. This is not a normal or healthy situation. We got this way from eating carbs as soon as we wake up – just like the Nutritionist told us to do. The mechanism to switch from glucose metabolism to fat metabolism doesn't work efficiently so instead of burning fat and maintaining a healthy blood glucose level, the body continues to metabolize glucose, resulting in an abnormal drop in blood glucose levels that cause us to feel lightheaded. We need food. Wrong! Actually, what we need to do is slowly retrain our bodies to efficiently switch into glycogen metabolism. Instead of eating carbs when we first wake up in the morning, eat a low or no-carb food like a cup of coffee (no sugar), pecans, peanuts, or almonds. This will help us feel less hungry and lightheaded. Slowly extending the time when we eat breakfast, will eventually enable us to make it all the way to lunch without eating carbs.

CHAPTER 6

MAINTAINING A HEALTHY WEIGHT

Another big challenge to extending our healthy, vibrant lives, is our body weight. Being overweight is unhealthy for many reasons, being both the cause of disease and the result of it. Gaining weight is terribly easy and most of us fall victim to it. It happens so slowly that we don't notice until it is there. Getting off those extra pounds is not easy, as reducing weight means reducing body fat. We never want to reduce muscle mass and we cannot reduce or change our bones, so it all comes down to fat.

There are over 90 different diets currently circulating and being presented as the best way to control weight and health. This is worse than the Tower of Babel. The cacophony of conflicting advice being thrown at people today is mind numbing and overwhelming. Most of these diets will help in the short term and may improve eating habits and health, but not one has been shown to be effective over the long term. It's interesting to note a study that compared weight loss and blood chemistry on several different diet regimes ranging from Atkins (high fat, very low carb, meat-based) to Dean Ornish (very low fat, high carb, plant-based), and found no significant difference! The conclusion was that almost any diet regime, that limited the intake of food, can result in successful weight reduction and an improvement in health metrics. The study was unable to quantify the long-term effects of the diets, but we have to conjecture that eating a high fat, low fiber, meat-based diet, as is done in Atkins, could have long-term negative health consequences.[38] Dr. Ornish, in a beautifully written review, where he compares his program with the diet developed by Dr. Atkins, makes the logical assertion that if calories matter in weight loss, then reducing fat intake must be an important consideration, since fat has more than twice the caloric content of protein or carbs.[39] In addition, the preponderance of evidence showing not only the benefits of fiber, but the negative consequences of a low fiber diet, predict that long-term, an Atkins regime will be damaging to health. Fiber reduces the caloric content of food and increases satiety, helping us to eat less. All good things. The study also notes that in selecting a diet, weight management is only one criterion, albeit a big one.

Eating too many calories, even for a relatively short period of time, can cause insulin resistance, the beginning of diabetes. What we eat and when are important, but even more important is how much we eat. The body has mechanisms for managing over-nutrition. The liver and muscles are designed to store surplus calories as glycogen initially and when the store of glycogen reaches capacity, to store the excess as fat. Having glycogen and fat storage is a good thing if the body is to survive not only periods of over-nutrition but also periods of undernutrition. When food is scarce, we can tap into the stored calories to maintain body functions. The brain and muscles especially need a constant supply of energy in order to function. The brain has little or no storage capacity, so it relies on a constant supply of glucose in the blood that comes from the liver and kidneys when food is unavailable. The muscles have their own storage capacity for short term and long term use in the form of glycogen and fat. When these are exhausted, the muscles use fat from other parts of the body or even scavenge protein from the muscles themselves. This is how it is supposed to work. But if we never experience undernutrition, then the fat is never utilized and only accumulates, leading first to weight gain, then insulin resistance, eventually to obesity and finally diabetes. Even skinny people can be diabetic because excess fat storage doesn't mean that they are fat. Actually, the visible belly fat is the least harmful of all. The invisible fat stored in the liver and muscles is the most damaging. Skinny people may not have a lot of visible body fat, but their liver and muscles may be storing too much fat. They are skinny/fat. To avoid storing excess liver and muscle fat, we don't need to starve, but we need periods of undernutrition (fasting) to allow the system to cycle like a battery, in order to maintain our weight and blood glucose control system in healthy condition. If the system never cycles, eventually it loses the ability.

The main problem with the popular diets is that in order to be simple enough for people to follow, they focus on one aspect of nutrition. For example: low fat, low carb, high protein, no meat, no white foods, no gluten, caveman, pineapples, etc., etc. I suppose if we ate only pineapples we might lose weight, but is that going to produces healthy results long term or be sustainable? Or eating no carbs as the Atkins diet proposes? Is that healthy long term or sustainable? There is an element of truth in all of these diets, otherwise they would not work for anyone. But clearly nutrition is more complex than just one factor. And to be effective, a diet should not be something we do for a few months, but rather a change in our eating habits that is sustainable for the rest of our lives, so that the benefits are long-term, not just to drop a few pounds and then go back to our old ways and regain the weight. This cyclic gain/loss/regain is the unhealthiest practice of all. We want a diet that we can benefit from and live with for the rest of our lives. We will not be successful unless we also consider the social and lifestyle factors, as eating is a social act and we may become outcasts by restricting our diet to foods that no one else in our social group is consuming. Our restrictive diet sets us apart and denies us and them the benefits of belonging to a family or a social group. Eating is about nutrition of course, but it is much more, and if we don't take these other factors into consideration we will fail long term.

The basic factors to consider in selecting what we eat are:

- Quantity (calories and volume)
- Composition (moisture, carbs, protein, fat, fiber, minerals and vitamins)
- Timing (time since the last meal)
- Balance (different foods that complement each other)
- Variety (eat lots of different foods)

Sorry. This is not as simple as just avoiding white foods! Good nutrition is more complex than that. On the other hand, we can identify some basic guidelines for selecting what to eat and when to eat, so that we can be successful in achieving a healthy diet that fits our lifestyle and social group.

We also need to keep in mind that there is much we do not know about human nutrition and diet. When the science is lacking, it is difficult to separate fact from the myth, the proven from the emotional, the truth from belief. The field is mired in emotion and beliefs with not enough science to dispel the misinformation.

> One of the most difficult things in life can be
> trying to put all of these things together.
> -Humpty Dumpty

We make approximately 220 decisions each day about the food we eat. In a lifetime, we will eat approximately 80,000 meals. These decisions matter, and in the long run impact our health, physical capabilities and lifespan. The World Counts estimates that over one billion people on the planet are hungry and that 17 million people die each year from starvation. At the same time, they estimate that over 800 million people on the planet are obese. It is ironic that starvation and obesity coexist to almost the same extent globally.

Food is a major contributor to disease, and as people in other parts of the world adopt a western diet, we watch the concurrent rise in the Metabolic Syndrome, where these diseases were virtually unknown before. The point is that the food we eat has a significant impact on our health and how we feel. The decisions we make about food selection and diet are not trivial and we make a lot of them every day. Making these decisions consistent with our lifestyle, can enable us to make these numerous diet decisions in a rational, consistent and expeditious manner that can save us from expending time and energy to consider each one separately. The problem is that we will not realize the impact of the decisions we make today until the consequences have accumulated for several decades. We don't want to wake up one day thirty years from now to the realization that we are overweight and unhealthy. How did that happen? How can we prevent it from happening?

Diet and Disease

The impact of diet on disease is a controversial subject with many unknowns. We are certain that too little of some nutrients in our diet will cause disease. Insufficient intake of Vitamin C results in scurvy. Too little protein will cause muscle loss. There are minimum levels of consumption for each nutrient, below which we risk the onset of disease, and there are maximum levels of consumption for some nutrients, above which there is a risk of toxicity. Clearly, we want to always be above the minimum intake in order to avoid the risk of disease, and below the level that causes toxicity. What is not so clear from the science is the level at which each nutrient is optimal for health, which may be many times higher than the level required to avoid disease. The optimal level is difficult to determine and there is significant disagreement in the scientific community.

It is well accepted, that to avoid scurvy, for example, we need a daily intake of at least 10 mg. of Vitamin C every day. The US RDA

(Recommended Daily Allowance) is set at 75 and 90 mg. per day for adult women and men respectively, to allow for a reasonable excess over the minimum required to prevent disease. There is evidence of benefit from consumption of up to about a gram per day, which is over one hundred times the level required to avoid scurvy. The point is that the optimal level of consumption for many nutrients is higher than what is required to prevent disease. In theory, if we are consuming a variety of foods, we will get at least the minimum amount of nutrients we need to avoid disease, but perhaps not attain optimality. This is where our awareness and intentionality come into play. If we want to achieve optimal levels of nutrients, we must intentionally modify our diet to include foods that contain those nutrients at high levels.

Atkins vs. Ornish

The Atkins and Dean Ornish diets are exact opposites, with South Beach and others somewhere in between. All these diets are attempts to provide a simple way to eat in order to reduce weight and improve health. They get some parts of the puzzle right and some wrong, but fail to achieve a holistic healthy, sustainable diet.

Atkins was right that we need to eliminate carbs in order to allow the body to switch into fat metabolism so that we can reduce stored fat and lose weight. There are benefits to doing this. But Atkins went too far. Eliminating carbs from the diet for days, weeks or more is unhealthy. In order to eliminate carbs from the diet, we must eat more protein and fat. Long term consumption of a high fat, high protein diet can lead to ketosis, kidney damage and other serious health impacts. Elimination or drastic reduction in carbs will also greatly reduce dietary fiber intake that is critical to establishing and maintaining a healthy and diverse microbiome. The bacteria in our guts, that produce so many health benefits, will literally starve on a low carb diet. And there are too many foods we like, such as bread, fruit and some veggies, that are excluded under Atkins, that it can make it difficult to stick to the diet long term.

On the other hand, Dean Ornish is also right that we can benefit from a high carb diet rich in dietary fiber and antioxidants. On the Ornish diet, the intestinal microbiome will flourish. High carb foods from grains and vegetables contain fewer calories and more bulk, making it easier to reduce total caloric intake and thereby achieve weight loss. The problem with the Ornish diet, is that it eliminates many of the foods we like or are culturally important, making it difficult to follow and adhere to long term. The best results achieved by Ornish were with people who attended his camps and strictly adhered to his diet regimen, largely because of calorie restriction.

How about we take the advice of both Atkins and Ornish? For fourteen to sixteen hours each day, much of which passes while we are sleeping, we follow Atkins, allowing our bodies to switch into fat metabolism with all the benefits of that regimen. Then for the other eight to ten hours, we follow Ornish and feed our microbiome with plenty of dietary fiber and complex carbs. This way, we get the best of both disciplines in a twenty-four-hour period.

Healthy Weight

Maintaining a healthy weight is important for a lot of reasons. Every excess pound of fat that we carry around puts stress on our legs, joints, heart, and respiratory system, in addition to retaining higher levels of toxins and causing inflammation. Being overweight is not good for longevity and not good for our health. Obesity slows us down, wears us out and will convince us that we cannot do today what we used to do. It reinforces the attitude of aging and death. We are all different, so it's not possible to define ideal weight without some study. Body Mass Index (BMI) is almost useless as it doesn't adequately adjust for body size and muscle mass. According to BMI Tom Brady is obese – no he's not. A better indicator is body fat content. This is not so easy to measure, but some trainers and clinics have the ability either through a scanner or a dip tank. We need some fat on our bodies to store calories and to regulate hormones. Women need a bit more than men for good health. Male world class athletes achieve body fat levels near five percent with women closer to ten percent. If you are not a world class athlete, fifteen to twenty percent is a reasonable goal. Any more than that is extra weight to carry around. We don't want to be there.

What was your weight when you were a young adult? Assuming that you weren't already overweight, chances are this is when you were at your ideal body weight and most healthy. How many pounds above this weight are you now? Most people have tacked on forty or fifty pounds since that time, probably all fat. Our bones are the same bones we had then. They have not grown bigger or stronger. Our joints are the same. Our heart and lungs are the same. Our muscles may have gotten stronger, but more likely are the same or weaker. Our body is the same body as it was back then, except now there is all this extra fat to carry around and support, putting extra stress on organs, muscles and joints. It's no wonder that we cannot do what we used to do. Calculate how much extra fat you are now carrying around and then go find a stack of books or a sack of potatoes or something that weighs that much and go walk around with it for a few minutes. The extra weight will instantly be noticeable and cause us to tire more quickly. This is what we are putting up with every day, except that the fat accumulated slowly so that we never noticed it. When we can take it off, we will notice it!

Nutrition is complicated and there are many factors to consider in a healthy diet. But there are a few facts that can put it into context. If we are above our ideal body weight, we are eating too much. Sorry – it doesn't get any straighter than that. We will have to eat less, if we want to lose some pounds or maintain an ideal weight. Buy a scale and weigh what your food in order to calibrate intake. We are probably eating more than we think. Too much 'healthy' food is not healthy.

It takes a little over 4,000 calories to make a pound of fat. If we overeat by 100 calories a day, in about two months, we can gain a pound of fat. This is really easy to do, because 100 calories are only a couple of chocolate chip cookies. Doesn't seem fair, does it? Exercise is very important for good health, but we will not lose much weight by exercising. The only way to control our weight is to control what we eat. Carbohydrates are a required nutrient – if we don't eat carbs we will die. However, if we eat too many carbs, we will get fat. The trick is to balance our carb intake with our physical activity level. If we are running marathons, we had better be eating big bowls of pasta every day, or we will literally starve to death. If we are a couch potato or computer jockey, and exercise for us is opening the microwave oven, then we had better reduce our carb intake. Reduce - not eliminate! We need carbs to live. How much? It depends on how active we are. Carbs are the fuel that our bodies run on. A healthy diet for a reasonably active person could include 350 grams of carbs per day. That sounds like a lot, but its only 1400 calories of the 2500 or so that we need in a day. The remaining calories are fat and protein. Our brain consumes about half of these carb calories, our muscles the rest. Any excess that is not consumed is converted by our liver into glycogen, where it is stored for rapid conversion to glucose when we need it. At some point, it is converted to fat for long term storage. That is the problem. Most of the fat we store, stays there forever and we keep adding more until we wake up some day with an extra forty or fifty pounds of blubber that restricts our movements, wears out our joints, makes our lives miserable, makes us unhealthy, stores toxins, and causes heart disease, inflammation, hormonal imbalance, hypertension, diabetes, cancer, and so on. All bad, no good. We don't want to be there, and we don't have to be.

It is worth emphasizing that the goal is not to be skinny! Too little body fat can also be harmful. Fortunately, most of us are at little risk of that ever happening! But consider the target of twenty percent body fat. Our 150-pound person, therefore, has a target body fat content of thirty pounds. That is not a trivial amount. If you ever saw a thirty-pound bucket of fat, you would be disgusted. The fact is that most of that thirty pounds of fat in the body is distributed around as thin layers that insulate, protect and lubricate our muscles and organs. It allows muscles to move freely, and protects organs from shock and damage. Fat absorbs hormones and moderates hormone levels. Fat is also a protective storage site for stem cells, which are important for repair and recovery. Fat has a negative side too. In addition to the weight it adds to our bodies, it absorbs and stores fat-soluble toxins and causes inflammation. Fat is an important part of our bodies and we would literally die without it. We don't want to eliminate fat, but control it. Fat is a good thing, but remember, too much of a good thing is often not a good thing.

Weigh yourself twice a week and watch out for changes. Don't obsess over it, but when you see a change, try to figure out what caused it. Keep cutting down on carbs and how much you eat until you start to see the numbers moving slowly in the direction that you want. When you get to your ideal weight, learn what and how much you can eat in order to maintain it. We need to enjoy ourselves sometimes, so when we go to a fancy restaurant, we should eat as moderately as possible, but we will likely overeat. Then we should compensate by eating less over the next few days to bring our overall diet for that period of time into alignment with our goal. There are no bad foods, only bad diets. This means that we can eat almost any food, as long as we balance the overall quantity of what we eat over a period of a few days.

One of the worst habits imposed on us as children, was the need to 'clean your plate'. Please don't impose this burden on your children or on yourself. Cleaning our plate will almost surely result in obesity at some time in our life. We need to stop eating when we have had enough. Enough does not mean full or sated. Eating until we are full on Thanksgiving is a tradition and certainly fun. But we don't want to eat like this every day. We need to learn how much we can eat in order to maintain our healthy body weight. When people tell me that they are eating Paleo, like cavemen did, I like to remind them that in order for it to work, they really do have to eat like a caveman. Cavemen and women did not eat three or more meals a day. They feasted when the hunt was successful and fasted or ate subsistence items like nuts and dried fruits until the next good hunt, which could be days away. Feasting and fasting may be the best combination. We can feast when we want to enjoy a really good meal, and then fast for a day or two to allow our body to digest, process, metabolize and clear out the waste, before another round of feasting begins. Fasting doesn't mean starving. It means reducing caloric intake for some period of time below the maintenance level, forcing the body to use stored glycogen and fat. The amount of feasting and fasting must be balanced to maintain a healthy body weight. When we feast daily, but fail to fast, the result is obesity and disease.

Listen to Your Body Talk

AC/DC got it right – we need to listen to our body talk. It talks to us with feelings, pleasure and pain. Thirst, hunger, satiety, exhaustion and many other signals give us a clue as to how our bodies are performing and what steps we should be taking to keep the body healthy. However, some of the signals can be misleading and need to be managed in balance.

Physical intelligence resides in our body. Our cells and organs have intelligence. In fact, it is possible that there may be more intelligence in our body than in our brain. As an example, Dr. Michael Gershon wrote a book on his discoveries about the neural processing capabilities that surround our intestines[40]. He estimates that there are over two million neurons wrapped around the intestines, controlling digestion and waste elimination for the body. That is roughly ten times the number of neurons in the brain of a fruit fly, and they can fly and do all sorts of annoying things. This is the second largest concentration of neurons in the body, second only to the brain. Did you know that your intestines were so smart? The liver is able to control blood glucose levels depending on what we eat and how active we are. It does this with limited input from the brain.[41] The brain is our main source of intelligence; however, we should not overlook the fact that there is intelligence in all parts of our body.

> When wealth is lost, nothing is lost;
> when health is lost, something is lost;
> when character is lost, all is lost.
> -Dr. Billy Graham

The first step in using our physical intelligence to help us live healthier, longer lives is to be aware of the presence of this intelligence. We are not used to thinking that our livers or feet are smart! But the fact of the matter is that these organs perform complex functions with little or no input from our brains. This means that they have an innate intelligence that enables them to operate and perform complex tasks. Our task is to realize this and learn to pay attention to it. Now that we know that our feet have intelligence, perhaps we can notice when they feel good or complain. Their complaints are not idle. The complaints that come in the form of pain or discomfort, contain information that could be very useful to us. Learn to listen and then respond with a change in behavior or shoes!

> If we don't change direction, we will end up where we are headed.
> -Yogi Berra

Obesity

The underlying causes of obesity include:

- Lack of understanding about nutrition and essential nutrients
- Lack of availability of fresh vegetables (frozen is a good substitute, canned not so much)

- High cost of fresh vegetables
- Lack of skill in preparing fresh vegetables in a palatable manner that people want to eat, especially kids
- Overnutrition, especially carbs (high carb foods are generally less expensive than high protein or fat containing foods, therefore people on low incomes often overeat carbs and become obese)

As we consider the nutritional properties of food ingredients, it is useful to measure or rate ingredients on the basis of the following criteria:

- Nutritional content (protein, fat, fiber, carbs, sugar, essential nutrient content, antioxidants)
- Availability (seasonality, knowledge and the existence of 'food deserts')
- Cost of the ingredient (per Kcal, per protein, per fat, per fiber, per antioxidant, per other essential nutrients)
- Convenience (preparation methods, waste)
- Knowledge (training, upbringing, cultural awareness and acceptance, recipes)
- Flavor (can be adjusted to local taste in the recipe)
- Texture (can reduce acceptance to novel ingredients, especially among children)
- Fun and enjoyable (includes foods served on Holidays, parties and special occasions as well as snacks, desserts and treats)

If we consider what kinds of education or intervention needs to take place to improve this situation, we can include:

- Nutrition education
- Awareness of novel ingredients
- Recipes
- Preparation methods

The causal factors of obesity center around a lack of awareness and can therefore be improved via education. There could be utility in learning how to develop recipes that combine ingredients to achieve an improved nutritional profile while minimizing the impact on blood glucose. This is a challenge that is not typically presented in cook books, even books purporting to offer 'healthy' recipes.

To be successful, a diet needs to provide a good nutritional profile, be affordable, available, convenient, good tasting, fit our lifestyle and be fun (sustainable and enjoyable)!

CHAPTER 7

MAINTAINING STRENGTH

Extending our healthy lives will require maintaining or enhancing several of our vital strengths: physical strength, immune strength to fight pathogens, mental strength, aerobic strength and circulatory strength. A commonly expected and accepted consequence of aging is a loss of strength. A leading cause of death, in otherwise healthy people, is loss of immune strength. When our immune system weakens, we can develop pneumonia and die from a common cold. Losses in mental, aerobic, circulatory and physical strength, cause us to reduce activity, which results in a further loss of strength, which causes a further reduction in activity, and so on in a declining spiral. We want to minimally maintain our strengths, but with some effort, we can actually learn how to enhance them over time. Don't settle for less! We must stay strong.

It's a great life, if you don't weaken.
-John Buchanan

Healthy Immune System

If we are going to be successful in extending our healthy life, we must maintain a healthy immune system. We suffer when our immune system is overactive or underactive. When we are younger, the greater danger is that the immune system is overactive, resulting in issues such as allergic reactions, autoimmune diseases and inflammation. As we age, the immune system function slowly declines, making us more susceptible to pneumonia, infections, the flu and food poisoning; events that a healthy immune system can usually handle. One way to slow or stop aging is to keep our immune system functioning.

The world is an eat or be eaten place! There is a constant battle raging inside of and on the surface of our bodies between the bacteria that want to eat us and the immune system that protects us. When the body dies, decomposition begins within minutes after the immune system stops functioning. Immune system function and failure originates in the intestines. Even though the intestines are inside of our body, they, and our skin, are the barriers between the outside world and our inner bodies. They isolate and protect us from toxins and bacteria in the food we eat. If we want to maintain a healthy immune system, we must maintain a healthy gut. We have talked a lot about the importance of a diet containing sufficient dietary fiber to feed and nourish a thriving microbiome in our intestines. A healthy microbiome is also important to maintaining a healthy immune function and is a significant factor in immune system failure and aging.

Inflammation is the most common and easily resolved issue resulting from an overactive immune system. Inflammation is basically retention of water in specific tissues as a response to damage. When there is real damage to a tissue, such as a bruise, insect bite, cut, infection, etc. the inflammatory response is beneficial to prevent further damage and aids in recovery. When there is no damage and the inflammation is persistent over weeks or months, the response is unnecessary and harmful. The effected body parts appear bloated, puffy, slightly red colored, tender to the touch and maybe even warm. Inflammation can affect any part or all parts of our body, including internal organs that we cannot see. Persistent inflammation is harmful and is often the result of a diet that is out of balance between foods that cause inflammation and antioxidants that fight it. Eating less of the foods that contribute to inflammation and more anti-inflammatory foods and antioxidants will help. It is also beneficial to take an antioxidant supplement every day. Curcumin and grapeseed extract are excellent antioxidants, and there are foods that we can make part of our daily diet to assure an adequate supply. I personally take a liposomal curcumin supplement every morning and have seen the benefits. My ankles are never swollen anymore. See the recommendations in the section on supplements in Chapter 3.

Autoimmune diseases are another destructive consequence of an overactive immune system. The immune system has been improperly sensitized and is actively attacking tissues in the body. These diseases are part of the Metabolic Syndrome that starts in the intestines with a leaky gut.

Allergic reactions are caused by an extreme sensitization of the immune system to a specific food protein. When exposed to this protein, the immune system identifies it as foreign and immediately launches a full-scale response that includes the production of histamines, swelling of body parts, rashes, hives, diarrhea, and vomiting. The most severe immune reaction is anaphylaxis, where the airway to the lungs swells and closes, resulting in asphyxiation and death within minutes. There are 138 specific proteins in foods that have been documented as causing an allergic response in a sensitive person somewhere. Please note that protein means a polypeptide, not the individual amino acids that are the building blocks of the protein. This is an important distinction. The incidence of severe allergies has been increasing worldwide for the past fifty years, but not uniformly. Peanut allergies in the US are common and rising rapidly, while in Asia this is not happening. Peanuts are consumed in both areas, but in Asia they are mostly prepared by boiling, whereas in the US boiled peanuts are rare and most peanuts are prepared by roasting. Does roasting change the peanut protein to make it more allergenic? Another interesting fact is that kids who grow up on farms in closer contact with animals have fewer allergies than city kids. Does exposure to more 'dirt' in the environment help to develop a healthy immune system? It is not clear.

Allergies to foods can develop later in life. Shrimp for some reason is a common food allergy that people develop in their fifties and later, even though they have safely enjoyed eating shrimp for their entire prior life. If we want to extend our healthy lives, we need to be aware of food allergies. Usually, sensitization starts slowly and then advances to more extreme reactions, until a full blown allergic response occurs. The early signals are mouth or tongue swelling, numbness or tingling, vomiting and swelling of a body part that came into direct contact with the allergenic material. If you suspect that you have experienced an allergic response, you can avoid exposure to that food again, which could be overreacting, as maybe it was a false alarm. Certainly, you should approach the suspect food cautiously next time. Take a small bite and wait a few minutes to see what happens before you eat more. If the reaction reoccurs, especially if it is more severe the second time, then you should stop eating that food and see an allergist to confirm. You don't want to risk having a severe or anaphylactic reaction. If you, or a partner have a severe allergy, you and they need to carry an Epi-Pen, which is a portable syringe with epinephrine in it. It contains enough epinephrine to slow the advancing severe allergic reaction in order to allow time to get to a hospital emergency room.

Celiac disease is an extreme sensitivity to gluten protein. It is now known to be caused by a sensitization of the immune system that occurs during a viral infection[42]. If a child is introduced to gluten protein while the virus is active in their system, they will develop celiac disease and be sensitive, often for the rest of their lives. The only solution is strict avoidance of all foods that contain gluten protein. Gluten protein is found in wheat, rye, and barley grains.

Immune Summary

Some steps that we can take to maintain and build the immune system include:

- Positive attitude
- Strenuous exercise and lots of activity in between
- Develop a healthy microbiome. A diet that includes lots of fiber to feed the microbiome. Beta glucan enhances insulin sensitivity and modulates the immune system, enhancing immune function when it is low and decreasing it when it is too high.
- Optimal levels of vitamins, minerals and antioxidants
- Sufficient sleep

Maintaining the Ability to Heal

As we age, the healing process slows down and eventually stops, resulting in death. The root cause of this slowing, is a limit on the number of times that cells can divide. Cell division occurs during growth, when we are young, and all during our lives as part of the healing process. When a cell dies, or is injured, a nearby cell divides to take its place. Leonard Hayflick in 1962, discovered that a normal human cell can divide a maximum of about seventy five times, after which it cannot divide further. This was an important observation, and the first evidence that there was a built-in mechanism that causes aging. From an evolutionary standpoint, it was thought that aging was an intentional process designed to limit the life of an organism. When an organism became "old" and no longer able to contribute to the group, it was beneficial for the rest of the group that this organism died. Later, it was discovered that the programmed aging was due to a structure in genes called a telomere, a section of DNA that resides on the ends of each gene, like a cap. The telomeres assist in the multiplication and separation of the genes that occurs during cell division. Every time a cell divides, the telomeres shorten. Initially each telomere contains about 25,000 DNA base pairs, but after seventy five divisions, the telomeres are shortened to around 5,000 DNA base pairs, and the division process comes to a halt. Healing, which requires that new cells be formed, slows or stops and death soon follows, when bodily functions can no longer be maintained.

Not all cells age. The reproductive cells in our bodies, bacteria and many animals do not age and are capable of dividing without limit. An enzyme called telomerase repairs the telomeres after each cell division, to maintain the original length. There is no shortening of the telomeres and no limit to the number of times the cell can divide. Our cells had telomerase to perform this function when we were young and large amounts of cell division were required for growth and development. After adolescence, the amount of telomerase drops rapidly, and the programmed aging clock starts ticking.

Telomerase is naturally occurring in some plants and is available as an extract for oral or topical application. No negative side effects have been reported in people taking these extracts in order to restore telomere length. In theory, this can restore the ability of the cells to divide freely and reverse the apparent age of a cell. There is a test that measures telomere length and estimates the 'age' of the cells in the body. Some people claim to have reversed the age of their telomeres by this treatment. This technology is available now, but is new, expensive and as yet, not fully proven.

There are several other ways in which we can improve and maintain our ability to heal. These include:

- Antioxidants: reduce or prevent inflammation, oxidative stress and damage
- Eat less: too much food puts a stress on the body. Managing the impact of over-nutrition, and the resulting buildup of fat and eventual obesity are all negative

- Exercise: any activity is beneficial by keeping muscles strong, blood flowing and burning excess calories
- Attitude: a strong will to live (life force) reduces stress, and gives us the reason to take the necessary steps in diet and exercise
- Stem cell therapy: Puts actively dividing cells (stem cells), harvested from our own body into places in the body where repair, and active cell division are needed

Maintaining Healthy Blood Pressure

Hypertension is another condition that coincides with 'old age'. Arteries may harden, the reduced flexibility of the arterial walls results in it more resembling a metal pipe than a living conduit that works with the heart to convey blood to the body. Partial blockages due to buildup of arterial plaque or calcium, will also restrict flow. These changes in the circulatory system will contribute to a rise in the blood pressure. But are these the real cause of hypertension? Dr. Thomas Cowan writes at length about the real causes of hypertension and hardening of the arteries in his book "Human Heart, Cosmic Heart"[3]. We already talked about his book and how blood flows due to electrical charge inside the capillaries. His claim that this is the root cause of hypertension and heart disease is a real eye opener. According to Dr. Cowan, the conventional wisdom that we have accepted, is wrong and the treatments applied today are only treating symptoms, not root causes. The result is that hypertension and heart disease continue to rage as significant risks to longevity. We don't want to go there. We need to learn from Dr. Cowan how to prevent the disease and if we already have the symptoms, how to address the root causes in order to reverse the condition. If we want to extend our healthy life, we must maintain a healthy blood pressure.

There is no evidence that high sodium or salt intake causes hypertension. If we don't have hypertension, eating salt will not cause it. If you already have hypertension, reducing salt intake will reduce blood pressure, so reduce salt intake. On the other hand, there is evidence that reducing salt intake, in otherwise healthy people, could increase heart disease. The best advice is to avoid hypertension and use salt moderately.

The root causes of hypertension, as best we know today include:

- Stress (number 1): Distress not eustress. Good stress (eustress) is energizing, healthy and not a cause of hypertension. Bad stress (distress) is severely damaging and debilitating on many levels. Sometimes the difference between the two is due to attitude. If you accept life's challenges as opportunities to be welcomed, these could create eustress. If you bear life's challenges as burdens, unfairly placed on your shoulders, alone in the world, with no way out, these same challenges will create distress. Worry is also a cause of distress. Some people naturally worry about everything, even those things that they cannot change or control. Attitude means a lot. Having a Plan B ready in case Plan A bombs, can reduce stress. Another option is to talk about our problems with a friend. Getting what seem to be insurmountable issues out into the open air can detoxify them or at least get them off our chest. Burying our problems and worries inside allows them to build and fester with predictably bad consequences. We are not an island or an Atlas carrying the burden of the world on our shoulders. Stress can be measured by testing blood for cortisol. Cortisol is a hormone that our body produces during periods of stress to enhance alertness and certain body functions, like increasing blood pressure and blood glucose level to enhance the ability to fight or take flight. When cortisol levels remain high due to persistent stress, there are many negative side effects, including hypertension and poor blood glucose control.

- Lack of sufficient sleep
- Lack of exposure to the sunlight and earth energy: Try to get sun on as much of our body as possible for ten minutes every few days. If this is not possible, radiant energy from a wood stove, fireplace, hot shower, sauna or hot tub can substitute. Walking barefoot in the grass restores our electrical charge, and feels great. Absorb earth energy into your body by doing Chi Gong. Take an earth energy pill (Oh – sorry, I haven't developed that yet!)
- Diet lacking in adequate vitamins, minerals, protein, essential fats, complex carbs, or dietary fiber. And predictably containing too much sugar.
- Imbalanced or underdeveloped microbiome: This is caused by diet and the factors we already talked about in leaky gut syndrome. The short chain fatty acids produced by the bacteria in our intestines are absorbed into the bloodstream where they clean up the high melting point fatty materials.
- Insufficient consumption of good fats and oils: We thought incorrectly for many years that saturated fats or cholesterol caused heart disease. We now know that a diet rich in oils from fish and nuts, as well as olive oil, safflower oil, sunflower oil, canola oil and even soybean oil will protect the arteries from the high melting point fats like coconut oil, palm oil, lard, butter and cocoa butter. Synthetic trans fats had even higher melting points, but these have been removed from our diets and are no longer a concern.
- Alcohol in excess
- Lack of exercise. Exercise is necessary, especially the kind that pushes the cardiovascular system to the limits.
- Insufficient hydration: we need to drink enough water to keep our bodies hydrated. This is actually a controversial topic because some think that excess consumption of water will dilute or wash out body minerals. I'm not sure who is

right! It's safe to say that we don't want to be dehydrated. And probably wise not to over-hydrate with too much water consumption. Balance!

There is evidence that a diet high in fiber and antioxidants will reduce blood pressure significantly. Cocoa powder and chocolate are especially potent. Proceed slowly as you increase fiber, monitor your blood pressure along with your blood glucose in order to observe how your body reacts. Like blood glucose, blood pressure needs to be controlled in a relatively tight range. Lower is generally better, to a point.

Avoiding hypertension will require many steps, many of the same steps that we need to take to avoid other ailments such as diabetes. The body is a holism and these ailments have a common set of root causes.

Exercise

Exercise and physical activity are critical to a healthy and properly functioning body.[43] The older we get the more important exercise becomes. Without exercise, we lose muscle quantity and tone. We need strong and flexible muscles in order to move, hold our skeletons in place, digest our food, keep our blood circulating and to breathe.

Dr. Otto Siegel, Genius and Longevity Coach, discusses the importance of exercising properly and not causing injury.[15] In our personal coaching sessions, he pointed out that the goals of exercise should be progressive:

- First to prevent injury (avoid what hurts and what you don't like)
- Second to preserve your existing capabilities (maintenance, no loss with age)

- Third to recover capabilities (get back to where you used to be, but lost due to inactivity)
- Finally, to develop capabilities (expand capabilities beyond where you are now or were in the past)

Lack of physical activity results also in obesity, hypertension, constipation, poor circulation, diabetes, and an overall malaise (bad attitude!). Let's start with a definition of exercise: exercise is repeating a motion in order to challenge a muscle or set of muscles. Let's differentiate between exercises that challenge muscles and those that challenge the cardiovascular system. Of course, our lungs and heart are powered by muscles, so an exercise that challenges those, is challenging muscles. If our cardiovascular system has good capacity, an exercise that challenges our legs may not challenge our heart and lungs. We need to pay attention to both. Any activity is good. Any exercise is good. Learn exercises that challenge various muscles and find ones that you can do enough of to challenge your heart and lungs. Start slow and increase intensity and repetitions as your strength and capacity improve.

The Canadian Air Force exercise routine is especially instructional on how to exercise. It starts out ridiculously easy, or so we think at first. For example; for pushups, it starts out with a few pushups done from the knees, which almost anyone can do, and requires that we perform just a few of these each day, then increase by one rep and continue daily. When we can repeat the exercise several days in a row, we add another rep, and so on for twelve cycles, at which point the intensity of the exercise is increased. After a few months, we are doing a respectable number of full body pushups, which of course was the goal, and it continues to advance in difficulty. The important thing about this program is that progress is manageable and therefore we don't hurt ourselves. If we do too much, or advance too rapidly, our body isn't ready and we pull a muscle or aggravate a joint. The exercise must stop for a few weeks or longer until it heals.

This is a good example of the tortoise and the hare – the tortoise will win this race!

Most people don't know how to exercise, thinking that for it to work it must cause pain. Then they avoid exercising because they don't like pain. Who does?! Pain could be an ache that indicates that a muscle has been pushed beyond its limit, resulting in increased endurance and strength once it has recovered. That could be a good thing. Or pain could be from a pulled muscle, or a damaged joint. While we are waiting for that pulled muscle to recover, we avoid any exercise that challenges that muscle. Meanwhile, that muscle and others nearby, atrophy from lack of use. The other problem with pain is that it may (and maybe should) prevent us from doing more exercise. That is not a good outcome. A better approach would be to find exercises that we enjoy doing and that don't hurt. We will find our strength and endurance improving, which is the idea. And as our strength increases, we will actually want to do more. Let's go there.

Any activity where the muscles are in action can be exercise. Walking is exercise. Stretching is exercise. Talking – is not exercise! We can build exercise into our daily routine and everyday activities. For example: when we take a shower, we can stretch and tighten muscles as we move to wash ourselves. It is amazing at how much of a workout we can get just by pushing and stretching our muscles as we move. It's a great time to do it because the warm water will help loosen up tense muscles, reducing the risk of pulling a muscle. Stretching is a great form of exercise that we can do often during the day. I love to stretch in bed. Every time I wake up during the night, and in the morning, I stretch my legs and back. Watch your dog or cat. Every time they get up, they stretch. Watch and learn!

Before we embark on any new exercise routine, it would be smart for us to get a physical checkup to make sure we are capable. The best way to do this today is to get a complete body scan. The price has come down to a few thousand dollars. The benefit is that it allows the doctor to assess our entire circulatory system to identify any blockages or developing blockages that could lead to a heart attack or stroke. Keep in mind that blockage of the arteries comes from at least two sources – fat and calcium. We can have low cholesterol and run several miles a day and still have a life-threatening arterial blockage caused by calcium deposition. The scan will also identify aneurisms, which are silent time bombs. There are many advantages to learning that we have a partial blockage of arteries. If the blockage is severe enough, a stint can be installed now to open the artery. If the blockage is minimal enough that no treatment is needed now, we can make lifestyle changes in order to reverse the blockage or prevent further advancement. On the other hand, if we get a clean scan, we have validation that whatever we have been doing is working – keep it up. We can relax mentally and get to work physically, knowing that our body can take the stress.

When we first start to exercise vigorously, it will hurt a little (good hurt), but after a few weeks the body will actually crave the work. The benefits to exercise are numerous and additive:

- Exercise builds muscle
- Muscle burns calories
- Muscles remove glucose from the blood, reducing blood glucose level
- Burning calories allows us to eat reasonably while maintaining a healthy weight
- Muscles look good!
- Muscles feel good
- Muscles build our confidence and improve our attitude
- Muscles help pump blood in the extremities
- Muscles hold bones in alignment and improve posture
- Muscles help move food and waste in the intestines
- Exercise improves insulin sensitivity
- Muscles improve our balance
- Muscles absorb shock from bumps and falls so we don't get hurt
- Muscles allow us to do what we want to do
- Muscles make you feel strong, be strong and feel younger

- Exercise builds endurance and improves circulation
- Endurance allows us to do what we want to do
- Exercise tires us so that we can sleep well

Two great books to read on exercise and diet are by Dr. Al Sears *PACE: The 12-Minute Fitness Revolution*[44] and Dr. Jeffrey S. Life *The Life Plan: How Any Man Can Achieve Lasting Health, Great Sex, and a Stronger, Leaner Body*[45]. In his book, Dr. Sears describes the fallacy of cardio training. Instead he shows how to use interval training techniques to challenge our cardiovascular system and muscles to induce real growth and improvement in capacity. It is strenuous, so it's important that we are physically able to handle it. If you are good to go, read the book and get to work. Interval training requires that we perform several repetitions of an exercise, getting ourselves to exhaustion as quickly as possible. We can do different exercises, but intensely enough to get to exhaustion within five minutes for each one. As our capacity increases, we will need to increase the intensity in order to get to exhaustion in five minutes or less. The first time I did this, I rode my exercise bike and got to exhaustion in a minute. Apparently, I wasn't in as good a condition as I thought! The good news is that when you challenge your body like this, it responds. I added fifteen seconds every few days and within four weeks I was up to five minutes of bicycle time. And I could feel the strength returning to my body. Personally, I don't like riding the exercise bike. To me it is painful and dragging myself to do it is a real chore. I have since found other exercises using small weights and a Bowflex® that I actually enjoy. The result is the same. I can push myself to exhaustion in a few minutes doing a strenuous exercise that I actually enjoy. What a concept! Experiment and find a set of exercises that you like to do and then use them to push your body to the limits. Go slowly and incrementally increase the intensity as you feel your body getting stronger and more capable. It is an exhilarating feeling. Make it fun and it becomes a sustainable activity we want to do every day for the rest of our vibrant, healthy lives.

One of the main reasons why we don't exercise is that we are not motivated. We can find a hundred reasons not to exercise now. There is always something else on our to-do list that must be done now. It is an example of the urgent pushing out the important. If we don't schedule the time to exercise, we probably will find ourselves tucking into bed, realizing that our good intention to exercise didn't happen, again. Sometimes, when I don't feel like jumping into a strenuous exercise routine, I trick myself to get started. "I'll just do thirty seconds on the exercise bike." When that is done, I can almost always convince myself to go another thirty seconds, and so on until I find myself at the goal. Easing into it slowly works. Having a routine also works, as we get used to doing it, and even crave it. And that is the bottom line – we must do it!

Roger Clements had a long, successful career as one of the top pitchers in baseball history. He attributes his success to many factors, and one is his unique exercise routine. He worked himself to exhaustion every day, and discovered that it was important not only to his physical health, but also to his mental and emotional health. Exercise produces endorphins, which give us a calm, good feeling all over. This feeling is good not only for muscles but also for our brains, and it reduces stress. Find a plan that works for you and then get good at it.

Another beneficial side effect of exercise, especially the high intensity kind, is the impact it has on blood glucose. When you start measuring your blood glucose often, you may notice that even a little bit of activity drops the level. That is the good news. A brisk walk, a few jumping jacks, jumping on a small exercise trampoline (my personal fav), even walking around while reading or watching TV is better than sitting. Look at how we have designed our work and our relaxation times – usually sitting or lying in a recliner. We couldn't have invented a more destructive lifestyle if we tried. We were not designed to sit around. We were built for movement. In fact, we were designed to run. An enlightening book on that subject is *Born to Run: A Hidden Tribe, Superathletes, and the Greatest Race the World Has Never Seen* by Christopher McDougall[46]. In the book, he analyzes the design of the human body and concludes that we were intended to be long distance runners. In fact, the reason our species was successful, was because we were designed to run and we were able to hunt by running prey to death. There is no animal on the planet that is capable of running the way we do, for as long as we can. We are running machines, sitting around idle most of the time. When was the last time you ran anywhere? We need to move and keep moving.

Living with Pain

Pain often is an unavoidable part of life. My father used to say, with his characteristic feigned lack of empathy, 'Enjoy the pain, when it stops you're dead!' Pain and pleasure are inseparable. Without pain, we would not know pleasure, and vice versa, but too much pain can cause the body to go into shock and even lose consciousness. Continuous pain is debilitating and exhausting, wearing down our energy and temper, but we cannot and don't want to completely avoid pain. We need to learn how to manage pain, accepting it when we must, while adjusting our behavior when possible. The first step is to differentiate between 'good' pain and 'bad' pain.

Good pain is usually muscle pain. If we haven't used a muscle in a while, the first few times we stress it, the muscle will give us some aching pain, stiffness or spasms. This is a good pain, because it doesn't indicate damage. The muscle isn't damaged; it is exhausted, sore and needs to recover. After it recovers from the stress in a few days, it will be stronger and better able to handle the stress. If we experience muscle cramps after increasing the intensity of an activity, first make sure to hydrate sufficiently and if that doesn't work, take a magnesium supplement to ease the cramps. We want to continue stressing this muscle in order to expand its endurance and strength, accepting the good pain as an indication that we did it right. This is growth.

Bad pain feels different, can occur anywhere in the body, and is an indication of damage. Bad pain is usually more than an ache. We may describe it as shooting, burning, or stabbing. We need to listen to bad pain, identify the cause and take action to remove the cause. Then we need to do what we can to help the body heal. This may mean avoiding whatever activity caused the damage. Bad pain requires our response. The body knows when something is wrong or when damage has occurred, and it indicates where the damage has occurred by pain. We need to listen, act and modify our behavior in the future. This is how we learn.

When my knee was hurting, I tried to relieve it of some weight and movement, which caused additional strain on my other knee and hips, both of which started to complain as well! When the intestines are in suboptimal condition, virtually every part and system in the body suffers, and we cannot see our intestines to assess their condition. That is why it is so important to listen to the wisdom of your body. The organs and parts send a signal when something is wrong. The hard part is recognizing and understanding the message. Pain is the most obvious signal and the easiest to recognize, but it is not the only one. Being tired or 'not being able to do what I used to do' are also signals. How often do we hear people say that? "Well, you know at my age its normal not to be able to do what I used to do". "At my age, it's normal to be in pain." Do we have to accept this as truth? Why are we putting up with it? Why aren't we listening to our body and supporting it so that we can do what we used to do or even more?

We want to avoid taking pain relieving drugs when experiencing muscle pain. Pain has a purpose, and muting the signal may allow us to continue the action that caused the pain and inflict further injury. Pain relieving drugs have negative side effects that are worse than the pain and will not be evident until years later. Some pain relieving drugs are addictive, even after only a few uses. I prefer to avoid pain relieving drugs unless I absolutely need them, and then only use them intermittently. Never take these drugs continuously or prophylactically. If I really am in pain and need a good night's sleep, then occasionally taking an over the counter pain medicine may be a smart move.

Avoiding activity may actually be the worst thing we can do when we are in pain. The body loses muscle tone and endurance in a matter of weeks. Many injuries, especially to joints, are the result of poor muscle tone. Avoiding activity will make it worse. We need to find an exercise that doesn't hurt the damaged joint in order to strengthen the muscles around the sore joint. This will help with recovery and prevent loss of muscle tone while we recover. We want to prevent spreading the injury to other parts of the body, as we avoid use of the hurting part.

If we are to successfully extend our healthy, vibrant lives, we need to learn how to manage pain. This means learning how to do the things we want to do without injuring ourselves. Perhaps we need to wear knee braces when we do strenuous activities involving the knees, for example. Maybe we need to learn what activities injure us and then avoid those activities or find an alternative approach that permits us to play and not get hurt. Over and over I have learned the hard way, that I have to experiment and find another way. When we get hurt, we need to learn how to heal ourselves. There are many kinds of therapy that can be useful including chiropractic, myofascial, acupuncture, massage, etc. Hot tub soaks and sauna treatments are also great for sore, stiff muscles. Experiment and find out which work best for you. Try everything, don't give up. We will need to be good at this!

CHAPTER 8

Maintaining Healthy Blood Glucose

Maintaining a healthy blood glucose level will likely be one of the biggest challenges that you will face in extending your healthy life. Failure to control blood glucose is called diabetes, but a multitude of health issues start long before the clinical disease state is reached. It is one of the most serious threats to a long and vibrant life, because it is pervasive, insidious, slow-developing, progressive, debilitating and ultimately deadly. Most of us are already exhibiting symptoms of inadequate blood glucose control, and too many of us will end up with diabetes. We must figure out how to prevent this from occurring. Doing so, will require that we make some changes, and the sooner we start the better. There are many interrelated factors that make solving the diabetes dilemma difficult. It will take some pages to unravel the details. Suffice to say for now that the solution involves diet and activity, but it is not so simple.

This is a personal story, because this is a battle that I also fight. I found, while researching for this book, that I was on the path to becoming diabetic and was already showing signs of being prediabetic. Denial was my first reaction. I checked my medical records for the past ten years and found that my fasting blood glucose level had been steady over that time at 118. This is not considered to be diabetic, and my doctor had never pointed it out as an issue, but based on what I was learning, this is not where I wanted to be. I began reading everything I could find, as well as testing my blood glucose often. What I learned from both shocked me. There are hundreds of studies that focus on one tiny part of the diabetes puzzle, identifying the root causes that gradually lead to the disease: excess eating, excess sugar, lack of fiber, and inactivity. But no one was putting together the pieces of the puzzle to create a comprehensive picture that would allow us to take steps to prevent the progression of the disease. I had a mission and a personal interest. I don't want to become diabetic. I want to extend my healthy life for as long as possible, and to do that I would have to learn how to retrain my body to properly manage blood glucose. I am happy to say that it is possible and I am doing it. Now I hope that I can help you to do the same.

One thing certain about diabetes, is that the disease is rapidly increasing. In 2015 there were 392 million people diagnosed globally compared to only 30 million in 1985.[47] The CDC estimates that in the US about six million, or twenty five percent of those who meet the clinical definition for having diabetes, have not been diagnosed. The WHO estimates that the extent of under diagnosis could be as high as fifty percent in some countries. Diabetes is the seventh highest cause of death in the US, reducing life expectancy by ten years. Diabetes is out of control, poorly diagnosed, poorly understood and likely to get worse because we are not taking the necessary steps to avoid it.

It is useful to understand that the body's ability to control blood glucose deteriorates slowly over time. It is a progressive disorder, meaning that the body progresses slowly from a healthy state to a disease state over a period of several decades. It happens so slowly, that we and our doctors often miss the warning signs and fail to take action soon enough. We are all on the path to diabetes, the only question is where we are on the path and how fast we are moving towards it. Unless we take action now, we will become diabetic.

There is uncertainty about what causes it – poor diet, obesity, age, genetics, lack of exercise, gender, lack of sleep, excess liver fat, intestinal microbiome imbalance and many other factors all contribute. The clinical definition is complicated and restrictive, resulting in failure to diagnose people early enough to enable them to take preventative steps. Instead, treatment is often delayed until the disease state is reached and drugs or injections of insulin are the only options. Diabetes and obesity are often observed together, with diabetes exacerbating obesity and obesity contributing to diabetes in a vicious cycle, but even skinny people can develop diabetes.

Additional complexity comes from the fact that there are several ways by which the blood glucose control system becomes compromised, that include: failure to produce sufficient insulin, insulin resistance in the liver, brain or muscles, overproduction of glucose by the liver, and failure of the liver and muscles to remove excess sugar from the blood. This complexity makes it difficult to detect, diagnose and to prevent.

There is a long chain of events that starts with diet and activity and ends with diabetes. But diabetes is not the end of the chain or the story. Inadequate blood glucose control is the first step in another long chain of health impacts that includes depression, physical capability and stamina, brain function, sleep disorders, obesity and finally other disease states such as heart disease, hypertension, stroke, kidney disease, cancer, and autoimmune diseases. Ultimately, if not controlled, high blood glucose levels can result in loss of limbs, eye damage and death.

Diet is a critical factor in developing and preventing diabetes. Chronic overeating, high sugar, and low fiber are the dietary factors that lead to diabetes. The foods we eat and even how we combine them into meals makes a difference in blood glucose control. We decide to have the salad and then drench it with high calorie dressing loaded with sugar and fat. We drink sugar-laden juices thinking that they are healthy. We rationalize that we can have that chocolate cake for dessert because we did ten minutes on the exercise bike this morning, when in reality the cake contains 500 calories and we burned 100! When it comes to eating, we do just about everything possible wrong. We have done this to ourselves. The problem is us, not the food we eat. We do not know how to avoid diabetes and unless we teach ourselves, most of us will eventually become diabetic. We have a lot to learn.

> People need to know that walking around the
> block doesn't burn off a hot fudge sundae.
> -Penny Kris-Etherton (Penn State University)

Our bodies, age, genetics, behaviors, diet, activity levels, etc. are different, making it important that we learn about ourselves in order to discover what works best for us. We will need to gather data, make observations and even experiment a bit to find what works best. A blood glucose test kit costs $25 and is easy to use. We will need to have one and use it to learn how our body responds to fasting, eating certain foods, exercise, etc. in order to enable us to learn what to do and what to avoid to improve our ability to manage blood glucose. A blood pressure meter is also cheap and easy to use – we need to have one and use it often, as the changes we will make to improve glucose control will also lower blood pressure. It has taken several decades for us to train our bodies to manage blood glucose the way we do today. If that is not working so well, then some retraining will be required in order to improve, and this will take time and numerous changes in our diet and lifestyle. It took us decades to get where we are. It will take a year or more to regain control.

Lastly, don't allow age or any other factor be a limit on what you can do. This is another fallacy perpetuated by our medical system today. If we are sixty years old and our fasting blood glucose level is 115, like mine, our doctor is likely to advise us that we are 'normal' for our age and there is no need to do anything. The normal fasting glucose level for a twenty-five-year-old is under 95, so why should we be satisfied with 115? Can we do something about it instead of enduring another decade of denial, while blood glucose control continues to deteriorate to the point that we will be prediabetic or actually diabetic? The answer is that we can do something now and we should not wait.

What is Diabetes?

The control of blood glucose and the factors that eventually lead to diabetes, are complex and interrelated. I will try in this section to explain these factors in as simple a manner as possible, but please understand that in order to make it simple, I must leave out a lot of the details. The details can be found in other chapters in this book or in the reference articles that I cite. If you want the chemistry and the details, please go to these articles, keeping in mind that the science is not yet completely agreed on. Even among the experts and scientists, there is considerable disagreement.

There are two routes to diabetes: a lack of sufficient insulin production and insulin resistance.

- Insulin is produced in the beta cells located in the pancreas. After years of high sugar intake, the cells wear out and fail to produce sufficient insulin, allowing glucose to build up in the blood uncontrolled. A catastrophic failure of the beta cells to produce insulin causes Type 1 diabetes. In Type 2 diabetes, the Beta cells are able to make insulin, but the amount produced is out of proportion to the amount of glucose present in the blood, allowing glucose to build up in the blood uncontrolled.
- Insulin resistance happens when the insulin receptor sites throughout the body become blocked or do not bind insulin efficiently. The result again is that glucose builds up in the blood uncontrolled.

There are many organs involved in the production and metabolism of glucose. When any of these become resistant to insulin due to prolonged exposure to high insulin levels over many years, the system becomes less efficient and fails to control glucose properly. Excess glucose accumulates in the blood because it is not being removed efficiently by the liver, muscles and brain, and the liver and kidneys continue to produce glucose even when there is sufficient or excess glucose in the blood. It is common that both issues exist: organs have become insulin resistant and insulin production has fallen to suboptimal levels, both due to excessive levels of sugar and insulin over many years.

Now, let's consider blood glucose level and define what is normal and what is diabetic or prediabetic.

Healthy Blood Glucose:

Healthy blood glucose levels range from 80 to 126 mg/dl. Anything lower is hypoglycemic, meaning too low and anything higher is hyperglycemic, meaning too high.

Morning Fasting Levels:

Blood glucose level should be lowest after an extended fast, as we experience when we do not eat overnight. Healthy fasting levels range from 80 to 100. The fasting level is a measure of how well your liver and kidneys are controlling blood glucose. If the fasting level is above 100, the liver or kidneys are not functioning properly. Test your blood several mornings in a row to allow you to learn about your bodies' fasting level. A big meal or dessert the night before could be the culprit. We will talk about the liver and steps to take to keep your liver healthy in a little bit.

Levels After Eating (Postprandial):

It is normal after eating a meal, especially one that contains sugar, for blood glucose levels to rise, peak and then decline again. If the peak level rises above 140, the meal contained more sugar than the system could manage, and therefore you should reduce sugar consumption in the future. If it goes over 140 after consuming a meal that contains a moderate amount of sugar and carbs, then insulin control may be the cause, meaning either that not enough insulin is being produced or the system has become insulin resistant. The only way to differentiate these possible causes is to test blood insulin levels after eating. This must be done by a doctor.

There is considerable controversy about where to draw the lines between normal, prediabetic and diabetic blood glucose levels. My interpretation and preference is to draw the lines lower so that we take action sooner. My suggestions are to define prediabetic and diabetic as:

- Fasting blood glucose between 100 and 125 is prediabetic, 126 or above is diabetic
- Postprandial blood glucose above 140 is prediabetic, above 200 is diabetic

The only test that we can do easily at home is for blood glucose. After eating a meal, test your blood glucose every fifteen minutes until the level returns to baseline. Watch how the level rises, peaks and then drops. Make note of the peak level and how long it took to drop. If it drops back to near fasting levels within 2 or 3 hours, the system is working. Peak levels above 140 are a sign that something is wrong, and the best response may be to change your diet to consume less sugar. If the level doesn't drop to below 100 within three hours after eating, again something is wrong. Try reducing sugar in your diet and see if the same pattern persists.

The Glucose and Fat Metabolism Model

When we eat a meal that contains carbs or sugar, the level of glucose in our blood rises, causing a proportional rise in insulin. Carbs must be digested and broken down into glucose before they can be absorbed. Glucose passes through the intestinal wall, directly into the bloodstream. The rate at which the glucose enters the bloodstream depends on how complex the carbohydrate is – basically how long it takes for the digestive system to break it down. Simple starches start to break down into glucose in the mouth as the food is chewed. Complex carbohydrates take more time to break down and may not be converted for hours or days, when the food reaches the intestines where there are bacteria capable of digesting it.

While blood glucose and insulin levels are both high, our bodies metabolize the glucose and we feel satisfied. After some time, our stomachs are emptied and the rapidly digestible sugars have been absorbed. The level of glucose in the blood drops. The insulin level in the blood drops as well, but not right away – there is a lag of some time, maybe thirty minutes, depending on many factors. When blood glucose level is low and insulin is still high, during this lag phase, we feel hungry. There are two possible routes we can take:

A. Our body is telling us that the glucose is gone and we need to replenish it – we feel hungry and we eat a snack or meal that contains carbohydrates. Our blood glucose level rises, the hunger dissipates and our bodies continue to metabolize glucose.

B. Alternatively, when we feel hungry, we can avoid eating or eat something that is low in carbs, like a glass of water, or some nuts. If we wait for the lag phase to end, our blood insulin level will drop and when at a sufficiently low level, our bodies will go into fat metabolism. The liver converts stored glycogen and fat into glucose and the hunger goes away even though we haven't eaten any carbs or sugar.

Scenario B is what we want to happen at least once a day. If we stay in scenario A, our bodies will not metabolize glycogen or fat. This is what happens when we eat carbohydrates several times a day. Some people even wake up in the middle of the night to have a midnight snack to quell the hunger they feel. This is the worst thing we can do. If we don't allow our bodies to go into fat metabolism, then we never metabolize fat. We're putting money in the bank and never taking it out. With money, this may be a good if miserly behavior. With fat, it is a disaster that results in obesity and disease.

This model predicts that in order to avoid insulin resistance, excess stored fat and obesity we should:

1. Never eat carbs late at night or during the night. If you must put something into your stomach late at night or during the night, choose something that has no carbs, like water or nuts.
2. Fast in the morning for as long as you can or eat a low carb breakfast like eggs, or nuts with coffee or tea (without sugar). By doing this we can extend the overnight fast for another four hours. The goal is to spend twelve to fourteen hours in glycogen metabolism.
3. Eat three or fewer times a day with little or no carb-containing foods in between meals.

We will find that to reverse the conditions of insulin resistance, excess stored fat and obesity, we will need to take more drastic steps.

Healthy Blood Glucose Levels

If you are already diabetic, you will need to follow your Doctor's advice and take the pills or injections that they prescribe. Failure to do so could kill you. Unfortunately, we don't know how to reverse diabetes once the disease state is reached. There are some anecdotal reports of success using herbs. Let's hope they are real. However; if you currently have healthy blood glucose levels and your body is able to adequately, even if not perfectly, control blood glucose, then you can benefit from reading this section. The steps we will discuss could prevent you from becoming diabetic in the future. It is critical that you learn how to do so.

I say 'learn' because you will need to test yourself to learn how your body is reacting to the foods you eat and to the activities you perform. Every body is different, so what works for me may not work for you. A fasting blood glucose test once a year during your annual checkup is only measuring one aspect of glucose management – how well your body manages glucose when you are fasting. Where did that glucose come from if you haven't eaten any sugar or carbs in twelve hours? It comes mostly from your liver, where stored glycogen is converted into glucose to keep your brain and organs functioning, even though you haven't eaten anything. A good fasting blood glucose level for a healthy twenty-five-year-old is about 95. When you are fifty years old your fasting blood glucose level might be 110. This means that your body is not managing blood glucose as efficiently as it did when you were in your twenties. This happens to people, when they don't do anything to maintain their ability to manage blood glucose. The other test that is useful, but more difficult to perform, is the A1C test. This test estimates the average blood glucose level during the past two or three months, by measuring the degree of glycation of hemoglobin in the blood. Sugar in the blood reacts with the hemoglobin via a reaction called glycation and 'sticks' to the red blood cells for months. The higher the blood glucose, the higher the level of glycated hemoglobin. Good values are reported as below 5.7%, prediabetic is from 5.8 to 6.4% and above is diabetic. If I dip you in two pools of water, one at 70 degrees F and the other at 130 degrees F., on average you are at a comfortable hot tub temperature of 100 degrees F, but you are dead. Averages don't mean much, when blood glucose is spiking too high, and the A1C will not catch it.

We are learning that many organs of the body are involved in glucose management, including the brain, pancreas, liver, kidneys, muscles, intestines and probably more. There are glucose and insulin sensors located throughout the body that stimulate the production of insulin, glucagon and incretins. Incretins are proteins produced in response to glucose in the intestine that stimulate insulin to rise even before it is absorbed into the bloodstream. There are receptor sites on the surface of cells throughout the body that insulin specifically binds to in order to enable the passage of glucose across the cell membrane, into the cell where it can be metabolized. When these sensors and receptor sites become insensitive to insulin, the ability to manage and metabolize glucose is diminished. This is how most of us get on the path to diabetes.

Insulin and glucagon are the two hormones that control blood glucose level. Insulin is the primary control, with glucagon level depending on insulin. In essence, insulin down-regulates blood glucose, preventing it from getting too high and glucagon up-regulates blood glucose, preventing it from getting too low. Insulin performs several functions in the control of blood glucose:

- Insulin promotes the absorption of glucose by muscles, the brain and the liver, removing excess glucose from the bloodstream. Decades of high sugar and insulin levels causes these organs to become resistant to insulin, meaning they fail to respond to the elevated insulin. Excess glucose is not efficiently removed from the blood, allowing blood glucose levels to rise out of control.

- Insulin shuts down the production of glucagon when blood glucose is adequate. When blood glucose drops, insulin drops and glucagon production commences. Glucagon stimulates the liver and kidneys to produce glucose, keeping the level of blood glucose constant. When the alpha cells in the pancreas, that produce glucagon, become resistant to insulin after decades of high sugar and insulin levels, the alpha cells continue to produce glucagon in spite of the rising insulin level that occurs normally after a meal containing carbs.[48] The result is that the liver and kidneys continue to produce glucose even though the level in the blood is adequate, resulting in high blood glucose levels.[49]

We train the system by the amount of sugar we put into it. An excessive amount of sugar overloads the control mechanism and eventually damages the system's ability to properly control blood glucose. The system becomes insulin resistant, meaning it takes more insulin to control the same glucose level. This resistance increases gradually with continued excessive sugar intake, until at some point the body cannot make enough insulin to control the glucose, with the result that blood glucose level rises uncontrolled. This is the diabetes disease state. This happens progressively, creeping up slowly and insidiously. If we know that our fasting blood glucose level is climbing, can we do something about it to prevent the onset of the disease state? That is the key question. If we want to extend our healthy lives, it is imperative that we maintain good blood glucose control. Diabetes is a debilitating disease with many negative side effects. We don't want to go there.

In order to learn how our blood glucose control system is working, we need to test our blood glucose level at several critical times:

- First thing in the morning when we wake up
- Fifteen minutes after we eat, repeated until the level drops back to baseline
- After exercising
- Whenever we feel hungry
- Especially if we feel lightheaded or dizzy.

We want to know what is happening to our blood glucose level and how well our body is managing it at different times of the day and after different activities. Armed with this information, we can start to figure out how to retrain our system to improve control. Here is what we want to learn:

- How well is the liver controlling blood glucose while we fast?
- How much does blood glucose level rise after a meal?
- Are there activities that drop blood glucose level?
- How low does blood glucose level go and when during the day?
- How high does blood glucose level go and when during the day?
- How long does it take for blood glucose level to return to baseline after spiking due to a meal?

We retrain our blood glucose control system by achieving low baseline levels of blood glucose and insulin. We do this by fasting. Avoid eating anything after dinner or between meals. Water is OK anytime. By morning, we have gone ten to twelve hours without eating. Blood glucose and insulin levels should be at baseline. Try to wait as long as you can before eating breakfast. You can drink coffee or tea without sugar. Or even a diet soda. Anything without carbs or sugar. If you feel lightheaded or dizzy, test your blood glucose. If it is below 80, eat some pecans or walnuts and retest in fifteen minutes. If it is still below 80, break the fast and eat some carbs. You don't want to pass out. The goal is to get your blood glucose level down to the low to mid 90s, by exercising or working while we extend the fast as long as we can. With some practice and time, you should be able to wait until lunch to eat carbs. And then for lunch eat a low carb meal such as a salad. For dinner, eat a moderate amount of carbs, in balance with your activity level. Remember – you need carbs to live, so don't eliminate them. What you want to see in your testing is that your fasting blood glucose level is in the 85 to 100 range. After eating a meal, it may jump up twenty to thirty points, and then after a few hours drop back down again. The less it jumps up after eating, the better. The faster it recovers back to baseline again after eating, the better. Ideally, your blood glucose level stays level all the time at or near your fasting baseline level, in spite of eating and activity. The more it spikes up after eating and the further away it gets from the ideal 85 to 100 range, the closer you are to becoming diabetic.

The Role of the Liver in Glucose Control

If your blood glucose level remains high or even goes up after a fast, it is an indication that your liver or kidneys are overproducing glucose. After using up all the glucose from the last meal we ate, blood glucose levels should drop, then after a short lag, insulin levels should also drop, signaling the liver to begin converting glycogen into glucose so that the blood glucose level does not drop too far. The brain must not be starved of glucose or we will get lightheaded and if the drop is extreme, even lose consciousness. The liver is supposed to maintain a steady level of glucose in the blood. If the levels after a fast are too high (over 100), then the liver is not functioning properly. It could be an indication of liver disease such as cancer, cirrhosis or Hepatitis.

More likely, it is an indication of excessive amounts of fat stored in the liver, called non-alcoholic fatty liver disease (NAFLD). The excess fat stored in the liver, interferes with the function of the liver. There is little known about NAFLD, how to identify it, how to prevent it, or how to reverse it. It is thought to be due to prolonged over consumption of food in general, and fructose specifically. The liver is supposed to remove excess glucose from the blood and store it as glycogen initially and then as fat, when the glycogen store is saturated. It also removes fructose from the blood, but as already discussed, it converts some of it to glucose and some to fat, without any apparent control. The problem occurs when the amount of fat in the liver becomes excessive. It can happen quickly, in a matter of weeks, or over a period of years. There is evidence that it can be prevented by maintaining a moderate food and carbohydrate intake. Drs. Mann and Chisholm[50] recommend forty to sixty percent of calories come from carbs. In a 2500 calorie per day diet, this translates to 200 to 300 grams of carbohydrates per day. If a person is overweight, they suggest reducing daily caloric intake by 500 calories below maintenance, which means to about 2000 calories per day, depending on activity level, in order to lose weight. They do not advise carb intakes below 130 grams per day, even on a restricted calorie diet.

The only food that has been clinically proven to reduce the excess fat in the liver and reverse NAFLD is beta glucan. Beta glucan is a soluble fiber found in oats and especially oat bran. It is also found in the cell wall of yeast and is available as a dietary supplement. George Inglett[51] with USDA developed Oatrim®, a concentrated beta glucan derived from oat bran and performed research on oat fiber to prove its efficacy in reducing stored fat in the liver and blood cholesterol levels.

Oat bran is a good food for breakfast. See Appendix 4 for the recipe. Eggs are also reported to be good.

Insulin Resistance

Insulin resistance is not well understood. The term is used to describe a prediabetic state, where insulin receptor sites located in the muscles, liver and pancreas can be blocked by the presence of excessive amounts of accumulated fat. These organs are supposed to store fat, and convert fat to glucose when needed, but when the amount is more than they can handle efficiently, the system fails. Insulin cannot bind to the cells to stimulate glucose uptake and metabolism, with the result that glucose builds up in the blood uncontrolled. High insulin levels are undetected by the pancreas and it continues to call for glucose production by the liver and kidneys. The liver and kidneys continue to convert fat into glucose even though there is sufficient glucose in the blood and glucose levels rise uncontrolled.

There are several ways in which the glucose control system can become resistant to insulin:

- The muscles become insulin resistant when excessive amounts of fat build up inside the muscle tissue. Some level of fat is normal and good, but not too much.
- The brain becomes insulin resistant. We don't know how this happens, but there is evidence that an insulin sensor in the brain triggers the central nervous system to control glucose production by the liver and kidneys. When this fails, the liver and kidneys overproduce glucose.
- The alpha cells in the pancreas become insulin resistant and fail to respond to high insulin levels. The result is the continued production of glucagon that stimulates the liver and kidneys to produce glucose in spite of adequate blood glucose.
- The liver becomes insulin resistant due to excessive amounts of fat stored in the liver with the result that it continues to produce glucose in spite of adequate blood glucose.

The excess accumulated fat in the liver and muscles happens in several ways:

- Eating too much over many years. Excess calories are converted into fat. The fat accumulates and is never removed.
- Too much fructose in the diet. The liver converts some fraction of all fructose consumed into fat.
- Lack of exercise. Every muscle stores fat that it alone will use. Any muscle that is not exercised sufficiently to use up stored fat, will accumulate fat to excess levels and become resistant.

Insulin resistance develops slowly over many years as the capacity of the system to respond to persistently elevated insulin levels deteriorates.

The Pieces of the Diabetes Puzzle

Our goal is to put together the pieces of the diabetes puzzle. First, we must figure out if we have an issue. We want to know where on the path to diabetes we are now, so we can take steps to prevent or reverse it.

The first step is to identify if we have an issue with blood glucose control.

1. Start by testing your fasting blood glucose level first thing in the morning, before you have eaten anything or exercised. Do this for at least five mornings. If the level is consistently above 100, you should go further to find out why. If the level is above 140, you should see a doctor. You want to do this test yourself, as the test performed at a clinic or doctor's office is delayed. The activity you perform in the morning before getting your blood drawn at the clinic is enough to drop the blood glucose level, giving a false low reading.

2. Test your blood glucose level before and after eating a meal. It's not necessary to eat anything special. Eat as you normally would and see what happens. Test your blood before starting to eat and then every fifteen minutes for three hours. The intent is to see how much your blood glucose level goes up after eating and then how long it takes to come down again.

3. Try some different activities. Test your blood glucose before and after exercising. Try different types of exercise to see what happens. I bought a 36-inch exercise trampoline and use it several times during the day, especially in the morning. Just two minutes of jumping around can reduce

my blood glucose level by fifteen points or more. This is fun and involves the biggest muscles in the body – the legs. The idea is to use your muscles to burn glucose and get it out of your blood. I find that strenuous exercise like stationary bike or lifting weights is even more effective at lowering blood glucose level and have seen my level drop from 130 to 92. I was happy with that! On the other hand, I notice that after I have successfully lowered my blood glucose by some activity, all I have to do is sit at my desk for half an hour and it rises back up again.

4. Test your blood glucose when you don't feel right. If you are lightheaded, dizzy, tired or even very hungry, test your blood to see if the glucose level is the culprit. If blood glucose drops below 80 mg/dl you are likely to feel lightheaded, dizzy or tired. Test it again in fifteen minutes. If it is still below 80, eat something.

5. Experiment with different foods, in different combinations. Make it a game and have some fun.

What to Do

If your glucose is always between 80 and 100, no matter when you test it, you are good and can focus on maintenance. If your fasting glucose is 126 or above, your glucose after eating a meal is over 140, or any single reading is above 200, see a doctor now. If your glucose is below these numbers, but above 100 after fasting, then you are prediabetic and need to take steps now.

1. Exercise of any kind is beneficial to reducing blood glucose. The more the better. The more strenuous and intense, the greater the drop. The idea is to use the muscles to metabolize glucose and remove it from the blood. The drop is temporary of course, but any drop is beneficial. Repeated exercise can

build muscle mass and strength, which increases the amount of glucose that your body can burn, even when not active. The benefit is cumulative and builds over time. Exercise is also known to improve insulin sensitivity, reversing insulin resistance for three to four days, which is why regular exercise is so important to managing blood glucose and reversing insulin resistance. Find exercises that you enjoy and do them often during the day. After dinner, take a walk.

2. Unless you are already thin, losing weight is also known to improve blood glucose management.[52] Obesity is both a cause of diabetes and a result of it. It is a vicious cycle that must be broken in order to get better. Obesity reduces the effectiveness of exercise, and certainly makes it more difficult to exercise. Excess stored fat changes your body chemistry, hormone levels and liver enzymes. Men need a minimum of five percent body fat to be healthy. Women need about ten percent body fat for proper hormone control. Most of us are nowhere near these levels, so not a worry. We should all aim for fifteen to twenty percent body fat as a reasonable and achievable goal.

3. Change your diet.[53] Start by eliminating as much sugar from your diet as you can. We do not need to eat any sugar. There is often sugar hiding in the foods you eat. Do you take sugar with your coffee or tea? If so, reduce the amount slowly until you no longer need it. Stop drinking sugar-containing beverages like soda and juices. There is no evidence that sugar substitutes are harmful or interfere with blood glucose management, so use them in moderation if you need sweetness. Yogurt, except the unsweetened varieties, often contains a lot of sugar, especially ones with fruit. If you eat cereal, eliminate the types with added sugar and don't add it yourself. Sugar is everywhere, so you will need to be diligent.

4. There is a lot of evidence that changing your diet drastically to a low or very low carbohydrate diet is beneficial to improving blood glucose management. The normal recommended level

of carbs in a diet is about sixty to seventy percent of caloric intake, which for a 2000 calorie per day diet is 350 grams. One study suggests that we should go back to pre-industrial levels of carbs, which they estimate to be 43% or 215 grams per day. A low carb diet contains about 130 grams per day, which is the minimum recommended by ADA. A very low carb diet contains 50 – 75 grams of carbs per day. Unless you are extremely diligent, achieving that level of carb intake every day will be difficult. It is more reasonable to aim for the 130 to 215 grams of carbs per day. However, to see any benefit may take over three months. This is why most people fail to see the benefit – they don't persist long enough or drop carb intake low enough. It's not easy and unless you are obese, probably unnecessary.

5. Chronic overeating causes oxidative stress, which causes insulin resistance, which causes NAFLD, which causes diabetes. This long chain of events obscures the cause/effect relationship between overeating and diabetes. Remarkably, a study by Knudsen showed that overfeeding combined with inactivity increased insulin resistance in healthy young men in only fourteen days.[54] The body has a mechanism for handling excess calories in the diet, initially storing the glucose that is not needed at that time as glycogen in the liver and muscles, but there is a limit. When the limit is reached, the next step is to convert the excess glucose into subcutaneous adipose tissue or belly fat. This is the biggest store of fat in the body. But again, there is a limit to the rate at which excess calories can be processed and deposited. When this rate limit is exceeded, meaning we are taking in more calories than the storage mechanism can process, the additional calories get stored as ectopic fat in the liver. The result of too much fat stored in the liver is NAFLD, insulin resistance and diabetes.[55] Chronic and persistent overeating is one of the biggest risks to our health long term.

We must eat less. If we eat less, what we eat becomes far less important. If any of the 90 or so popular diets did any good at all, it was in helping people eat less calories.

6. Fasting is an excellent practice to recalibrate the blood glucose control system and improve insulin sensitivity. The goal is to avoid solid food for some period of time so that there is no sugar, carbs, fats or protein entering the bloodstream. We need to continue to drink liquids even when fasting so as not to dehydrate. Make morning fasting a part of your daily regimen as a great way to reduce overall daily caloric intake to help control weight. Do a twenty-two hour fast once a week to push your control system into fat metabolism. See the section on glucose management for a full discussion of the benefits of fasting on fat metabolism. Fasting will be found to be highly beneficial in prevention and perhaps reversal of insulin resistance and diabetes.

7. Now I'm going to tell you the opposite about diet! Eliminating sugar or changing to a low or very low carb diet are difficult to achieve consistently for a sufficient time to have an impact. For lasting impact, you will have to make these changes for the rest of your life. Most of us are not willing or able to make that kind of commitment. And there is even good reason not to make these drastic changes. By eliminating fruit and sugar-containing vegetables from our diets, we reduce our quality of life and also eliminate beneficial nutrients and vitamins. Remember the chapter on life force? Living without bananas, strawberries, oranges, chocolate chip cookies and donuts will not be fun and will weaken your life force. This could be detrimental to your health. In light of this realization, here are two points to consider: First, unless you are willing to go extreme in eliminating sugar and going low carb long term, what you eat is not going to matter very much. The fact is that how you process what you eat is more important than what you eat, and this depends on the health of your

microbiome, your activity level, whether you are insulin resistant or not and whether you are producing sufficient insulin or not. Secondly, there are other ways to manage blood glucose that are not so demanding. And finally, by eliminating whole groups of foods from our diets, we may unwittingly cause the next wave of diseases and not know it for thirty years. I suggest that you eat the foods you like, reducing sugar consumption as much as possible, while still enjoying fruits and snacks in moderation. Then, focus on the other steps that you can take to manage blood glucose such as exercise, eating less, losing weight, periodic fasting, increasing fiber intake, adding some new items to your diet, etc. You are more likely to stick to a moderate approach and therefore more likely to be successful.

8. Add some new things to your diet. There is some evidence that the following foods can be beneficial.

    a. Dietary fiber – There are a lot of benefits from increasing dietary fiber intake and improved blood glucose control is one. Fiber produces short chain fatty acids, increases the viscosity of food in the digestive system, allows more time for bacteria to ferment excess sugar, slows absorption of sugar into the blood stream[56], reduces the permeability of the intestinal wall (leaky gut), and more. Americans consume about 11 grams of fiber per day. The USDA Guidelines for Americans now says we need over 30 grams per day. Some recommend that we need between 50 and 100 grams a day. Fiber and exercise are the two most important elements in blood glucose control and health overall.

    b. Oat bran – oat bran contains beta glucan, a beneficial dietary fiber that has been clinically shown to reduce the amount of fat stored in the liver and improve insulin sensitivity. Beta glucan can also be derived from yeast cell walls and is available in convenient 500 mg capsules. This is a game changer. Take it every day. Almost all of us have an excess amount of fat stored in our liver, which is the cause of fatty liver disease and liver dysfunction in blood glucose control. You will also see and feel the benefits in your digestive system.

c. Vitamin D3 – has been shown to be important in glycemic control and prevention of diabetes.[57] We should be getting Vitamin D from exposure to the sun, but most people don't get enough. You need to take a supplement of 6,000 IU twice a day. Have your blood tested to assure that you are near the top of the 30-100 ng/ml recommended range.

d. Vinegar – take an ounce of vinegar a day. Put it on a salad, dip bread into it, mix it into a beverage (yuk) or if you're really tough, sip it! Make it part of your meals. Cider vinegar, especially the unfiltered kind is supposed to be the best, but Balsamic is great too.

e. Fenugreek seed – take a teaspoon a day (three – four grams) of powdered fenugreek. It is a good source of fiber too. I add it to my oat bran cereal.

f. Cinnamon – add a little to something that you eat. I add it to my oat bran cereal every morning.

g. Antioxidants[58] – have many benefits in our diet including: slowing aging, reducing inflammation, neutralizing free radicals, eliminating AGEs (Advanced Glycation End products) from the body, preventing cancer and improving blood sugar control. All antioxidants are good and you want to include several in your daily diet. Curcumin (also called turmeric spice) is one of the best. The spice itself is good, but the prepared versions are far more potent. The best is the liposomal form, which is highly absorbable by the body. Cocoa powder, ground cinnamon are also powerful antioxidants that are easy to incorporate into your daily diet, but be careful not to overdo it. Two tablespoons of cocoa powder a day is good. A teaspoon of ground cinnamon a day is good too. Grapeseed extract and lutein are available as capsules. There are other good antioxidant foods that you may like, but are a little rough, such as ginger and cloves. Coffee, tea, and red wine are also good. The idea is to incorporate a little of each into your daily diet in order to get enough antioxidants. If you have inflammation of your ankles, arms or face, you likely need more antioxidants. If you like to analyze your diet, look up the ORAC value of the foods you eat. It stands for Oxidation Radical Absorbance Capacity and is a measure of the amount of free radicals that a material can neutralize, which is what antioxidants do.

    h. Milk Thistle Oil and Powder – reported to detoxify the liver.

9. There are also some things to avoid in order to improve your blood glucose management. There is no evidence that sleep improves blood glucose control, but a lack of adequate sleep will likely make it worse. Likewise, stress is harmful. Alcohol in excess is also a stress on the liver to avoid.

When you put all the pieces together, it creates a complex and not so surprising picture. Exercise, fasting, good diet, eating less calories, losing weight if indicated, increased dietary fiber, antioxidants, keeping hydrated, getting adequate sleep and avoidance of stress. Those are all good things to do in any case. Why wait until we develop indications of being prediabetic? Start now.

Summarizing the Diabetes Scenario

1) The path to diabetes

- Blood glucose is one of the most tightly controlled materials in the body, with very good reason. Too much glucose or too little, both have severe health consequences, so tight control is critical. Only about 4 grams of glucose are circulating in our blood at any one time. This is less than a teaspoonful.
- Just about everything has an impact on blood glucose control, and blood glucose control has an impact on just about every system in the body. The body truly is a holism. When blood glucose control is out of balance, everything is out of balance and the consequences are manifest and extensive throughout the body. Adequate blood glucose control is critical to our vibrant, extended health.
- High levels of glucose stress the ability of the system to control it in the blood.
- Failure to adequately control blood glucose results in high levels of glucose in the blood, further stressing the system.
- Control progressively declines until the disease state is reached.

2) The main factors in causing diabetes

- There is considerable scientific evidence that diabetes is caused by the confluence of three main factors over many years:

    i) Poor condition of the intestine, especially a compromised mucosal layer and a depleted, imbalanced bacterial population
    ii) Chronic overeating, and high sugar consumption
    iii) Lack of physical activity, especially challenging cardiovascular exercise

3) Diet and Diabetes

- Blood glucose control starts with the food we eat. When the systems are functioning properly, we can literally eat anything and process it efficiently and safely. But the stress we put on the system by chronic overeating and high sugar intake, eventually degrade the ability of the system to adequately control blood glucose and we start on the path to diabetes.
- Limit the amount of sugar
- Increase consumption of complex carbohydrates and fiber
- Balance the amount of protein and fat in a meal
- Select the combination of foods in a meal to minimize blood glucose spikes
- Select the combination of meals to create a diet that controls calories and nutrients
- Be aware of the long term accumulated impact of what we eat
- Fast fourteen hours, three to five days a week (eat two meals a day)
- Fast twenty-two hours, once a week (eat one meal a day)

4) Exercise intensely to exhaustion 3 times a week

5) Add Good Stuff to Your Life

(1) Antioxidants (Curcumin, cocoa, cinnamon, whole grains)
(2) Vitamin D3 (6000 IU twice a day)
(3) Vinegar (20 ml once or twice a day)
(4) Eat fermented foods such as yogurt, kefir, kombucha, and sauerkraut

I hope this scenario begins to point towards a solution to diabetes. We may not be able to reverse the disease state, but at a minimum we can take steps long before progressing there to avoid diabetes.

CHAPTER 9

MANAGING THE
AGING PROCESS

We have considered many factors that contribute to aging and what we can do to slow, stop or even reverse these factors. The perspective we want to develop is that there is an opportunity to balance and optimize each one. The result of too little of one or too much of another is imbalance, a failure to optimize the benefits. Too much of something is often as harmful as too little. The optimal amount of each depends on many things, including the uniqueness of our own bodies, our activities, our attitude, our environment and many other criteria. Optimizing one factor is powerful. Optimizing many factors is life-changing. It is wrong to oversimplify, or prescribe based on the average, as most diet and self-help books do. It is risky to extrapolate from incomplete data and correlations to recommended practices and avoidance diets, as some experts do. We must learn about the factors, assess, and then based on our unique situation, do what is optimal for us.

To summarize the main points that we have discussed in this book, here are some factors to consider in our quest for a longer, healthier, vibrant life:

Diet and Nutrition:

- Body weight management – what is the scale indicating? How much body fat do we have?

- Balancing carb intake with activity level
- Fasting for twelve to fourteen hours at least three days a week (this means eating two meals)
- Fasting twenty-two hours once a week (this means one meal that day)
- Getting an optimal level of vitamins and minerals (not minimal to prevent disease, but sufficient to optimize health)
- Getting 50 grams a day of fiber every day
- Getting at least ½ gram a day of Beta Glucan every day
- Getting sufficient antioxidants to prevent inflammation

Exercise:

- Exercising to exhaustion to develop strength and endurance
- Exercising too little or too much (less than three days a week is too little, more than five days a week is likely too much unless you are a serious athlete)
- Allowing the body to recover in between sessions
- Constantly pushing to achieve higher levels – incrementally, slowly like the Canadian Air Force regimen
- Seeing the benefits, especially endurance and strength
- Exercising properly, good technique, good equipment, etc.
- When was the last time you ran?
- Physically capable of doing what we want to do
- Improving, staying the same or gradually losing strength and endurance
- If we stay on the path we are on now, where will we be physically in ten years, twenty years, or even fifty years?

Attitude:

- Attitude mostly positive
- When we get into a bad mood, how long do we stay there?
- How often do we get into bad moods?
- How do we get out of a bad mood?
- How is our walking posture? Do we look at the ground most of the time or all around?
- When was the last time we skipped just for joy?
- Do we use essential oils to stimulate our parasympathetic nervous system?
- Do we feel stressed? What is our cortisol level?
- Do we get 'upset' when things go wrong? Does it help us or anyone else, when we get 'upset'? How is that working for us? It is a choice.
- Do we enjoy our life? Do we love our life? Do we love ourselves? If not, why not?
- Do we want to live another fifty years as we are now? What changes do we need to make?

Breathing:

- Practice deep, full lung breathing at least twice a day for a minute or more
- After deep breathing, do we feel more relaxed?

Hydration:

- We need water to live even more than food. Only air is more urgent. How much is enough? How much is optimal? I leave this to you to research - Homework!

Reflection, thinking

- Reflection is good as long as we don't get stuck in the past. The past was what it was and we should enjoy it and reflect on it occasionally. After all there are some great experiences there that we want to enjoy. Thinking is actually a skill that we can practice to get better at. We can benefit from some five-year-old questioning and wondering about it all. I enjoy asking Siri questions when one pops into my head. What is the normal body temperature of a vulture? And does its high body temperature allow it to eat dead stuff and not get sick? Hmm…

Reading

- What are we reading? It will impact our attitude and mood. I suggest a well-rounded range of topics to keep us thinking and on our toes.
- Go back and read or re-read some of the classics. Maybe my life experience has changed my perspective, allowing me to appreciate them more the second time. Some of my favorites include: Frankenstein by Mary Beth Shelly (the original – it is an elegant and intellectual story); Moby Dick by Herman Melville; War and Peace by Tolstoy; anything by Dostoevsky, Hemingway, Steinbeck.
- Are we reading what I call 'crazy' books that can expand our mind? I've referenced a few already, like *Lab Girl* by Hope Jahren[21], and *Living without Death* by James Strole and Bernadeane[1]. Here are a few more that are bound to bring about a mood change!: *Life* by Keith Richards[59]; *Honey from a Weed* by Patience Gray[60]; *Just Getting Started: Fifty years of living*

FOREVER, Insights on agelessness and immortality [61] by James Strole and Bernadeane, with Joe Bardin; *Infinite Jest* by David Foster Wallace[62]; or *Shamanic Reiki: Expanded Ways of Working with Universal Life Force* by Llyn Roberts and Robert Levy[63].

Working

- Work is such an important part of our lives and our identity. Whether we are just starting out or retired, we need good work to do. The biggest mistake we make is looking for the perfect job or my favorite – "work that we enjoy". Good luck with that! Work is, after all, a four-letter word! There are no perfect jobs and even the best jobs and bosses have their bad moments. Flip it around! If we want to succeed, we need to enjoy the work we are doing instead of looking for work that we enjoy. We will be a lot happier and more likely to be successful instead of miserable. It is a choice! Once again, attitude is critical.

- The happiest people have work to do and do it well. Ever wonder why successful rich people keep working? It's not about the money. It's about the satisfaction from working hard and being successful. Success against a respectable challenge is a reward far more powerful and satisfying than money.

Dreaming

- Dreaming by its nature is forward looking and optimistic. If we want to extend our healthy lives, we need to keep dreaming, learning, planning, and of course doing.

Sleep and Relaxation

- We all have different requirements for sleep. The key is to know your body and give it the sleep that it needs, when you can. And when we cannot, compensate by taking naps or resting when we can. The biggest mistake is to wait until the weekend, or until vacation to catch up. The best advice is to take care of ourselves every day.

- Relaxation doesn't have to mean sitting in a chair watching TV. It also doesn't have to mean lying in a beach chair all day. Sleep and relaxation are like required nutrients; our bodies don't have any ability to store excess today for use in the future. We must have the minimum daily requirement today or accept the consequences.

Stem Cells

- Stem cells – still new but the technology is being practiced with reportedly excellent results for many diseases and ailments. The concept is simple: harvest your own stem cells from belly fat (we all have plenty of that), grow them to increase the number, inject them into the body where repair is needed and finally, store them for future use. The cells that are harvested and stored now are going to be younger and more active than the cells in our body will be in ten years when we may need them for some issue, so it is prudent to act now, even if we don't need the treatment now.

Other Stuff

- There is an awful lot of other stuff out there to consider regarding life extension and health, that is beyond the scope of this book, or perhaps any book. Technology is advancing rapidly and impactful discoveries will be made soon. We will need to observe, experiment and learn how to use what is available in order to extend our healthy, vibrant life.

Those who dream with their eyes open are dangerous people, as they work in the daylight to make their dreams come true.
-Alexander Pope

Attitude

I started this book talking about the importance of attitude, and now I am going to end the book on that subject. Attitude is extremely important in extending our healthy lives. A vision of what we hope to achieve is the basis of our attitude. If I can visualize living for another fifty years or even one hundred years, and keep that vision in mind every day, it can change my attitude about today and how I behave. Knowing that I have a future changes how I act today. That is worth repeating – I have a future! And because I have a future, I will take on bigger and more adventurous projects, perhaps even ones that will take many years to accomplish. Good! I will think about taking extreme care of myself today and every day so that I will be healthy and vibrant into that future. Good! I will look differently at how I spend my time today, perhaps more focused on achieving some goal, but also including some time to enjoy life. Good! It will likely change the way I plan my life. What is meaningful activity? What is wasting time? Am I learning? Am I reading and expanding my horizons? The answers to these questions will change dramatically if I have a future vision in mind to guide me. All good!

> The great French Marshall, Louis-Hubert-Gonzalve Lyautey walked thru his garden one morning with his gardener. He stopped at a certain point and asked the gardener to plant a tree there the next morning. The gardener said, "But the tree will not mature for one hundred years". The Marshall replied "In that case you had better plant it this afternoon."
> -John F. Kennedy

The point is that there is no time to lose. Let's use our time wisely and not waste it on frivolous or useless activities. Let's take time to build, develop, contribute, support and nurture our life force in order to enjoy and love life more fully. The world is a beautiful place, if we take time to discover and see the beauty. While I was writing this, outside my window were a pair of Cardinals, sitting on a branch next to each other. It was springtime, so the birds were courting and building nests. The male Cardinal flew down into the grass and picked up something, returned to his mate and transferred whatever gift he had found from his beak into hers. Life is so beautiful. Let's take time to notice and appreciate it.

> Whatever you can do or dream you can, begin it.
> Boldness has genius, power and magic in it!
> -Goethe

The Final Word

I've tried to hit the most impactful topics, but a lot depends on us. We are all different and what is impactful for you may be different. Extending our healthy lives will take learning and experimenting. Make it a goal to change or learn one little thing every week. It could be a new exercise, a new ingredient we use in our diet, a new Yoga pose, a new friend, or catching up with an old one. We are pushing the envelope as we move into the unexplored and uncharted territory of healthy life extension. We are in many ways, the modern version of explorers, embarking on an unpredictable journey of adventure and discovery. Our lives are literally at stake. The world could be flat and we might fall off the edge, like some experts have warned us. Or maybe they are wrong, and the world is round and we will find a new world of opportunity on the other side of the seemingly endless ocean of obstacles. Who knows what possibilities we will find on the other side of the horizon? A journey of one thousand miles begins with a single step. Let's take that first step, then go on to discover the many steps we can take to live a healthy, vibrant life, for as long as we dare!

APPENDIX 1

Recipe – Special Salad Meal
1/11/15 Len Heflich

Who says that you cannot eat a salad for dinner?

Well here is a salad that will fill you up and satisfy you as well as provide some great nutrition, flavor and texture. You will enjoy eating this as a meal.

Special Salad Meal

Ingredients:

30 grams (1 cup)	Arugula or other salad
110 grams (1/2 fruit)	Avocado
3 grams (1/2 teaspoon)	Cinnamon Ground
3 grams (1/2 teaspoon)	Ginger ground
10 grams (2 tablespoons)	Pine Nuts
25 grams (3 tablespoons)	Almonds (diced)
25 grams (3 tablespoons)	Sunflower seeds
30 grams (2 tablespoons)	Walnut Oil
100 grams (1/2 cup)	Papaya (cubed)
25 grams (2 tablespoons)	Pomegranate seeds
40 grams (3 tablespoons)	Balsamic vinegar
401 grams TOTAL	

Preparation:

- Place the arugula or salad green in a large bowl.
- Add the avocado, Cinnamon, Ginger, Chia seeds, Pine nuts, Sunflower seeds, diced Almonds, Papaya, Pomegranate seeds and then drizzle the walnut oil and balsamic vinegar over the top. If you cannot get papaya, you may substitute mango (available frozen), watermelon, bananas, cantaloupe or blueberries. You can be creative based on availability and season.
- Check that the sunflower seeds, pine nuts and almonds are not rancid. Rancidity is easy to detect – just open the bottle or bag and take a quick sniff. If it smells like paint, it is rancid. Low levels of rancidity are not harmful, but tastes terrible. Store the nuts and sunflower seeds in the freezer to make sure.
- I like to cut across the salad to reduce the size of the arugula and to mix in all the ingredients.
- It's fast, it will fill you up, it doesn't heat up the kitchen and it is very nutritious.
- Ready!

Nutritional Profile – Special Salad:

	Weight (grams)	Calories	Protein (grams)	Total Fat (grams)	Saturated Fat (grams)	Omega-3 (grams)	Cholesterol (mg)	Total Carbs (grams)	Sugar (grams)	Fiber (grams)	Sodium (mg)	ORAC (umol TE)
Totals	401	924	15.2	78.6	7.7	3.3	0	51.3	19.0	19.3	38.2	14,513

Summary: this recipe is high in protein, good fats, omega-3 fats, fiber and ORAC. It is low in cholesterol, and sodium. At 401 grams, total weight it will fill you up and it tastes great. Can you believe it – this recipe contains almost 20 grams of fiber? It's a great start towards reaching the goal of 50 grams of fiber per day. Your microbiome will love you!

January 11, 2015 L. Heflich

APPENDIX 2

A few comments are appropriate and necessary about this list. First, it is taken directly from the USDA Database, so not every food is represented, only the most common. For example; foods and ingredients like psyllium husk, and polydextrose are not on the list, and are useful in your diet, as these are 90% fiber, higher than any other food. Second, many of the foods that are highest in fiber are spices. These are good to use and incorporate into a diet for flavor, fiber and antioxidants, but since we cannot tolerate high amounts of these, individually they cannot be significant contributors of fiber. However; a little of several spices, used in different meals, adds up.

TOP 100 FIBER-CONTAINING FOODS (1 - 50)

USDA Nutrition Database

	Shrt Desc	%		%	%	%
		Water	KCAL per 100 gm	Protein As Is	Fat As Is	D. Fiber As Is
1	MUSHROOMS,OYSTER,RAW,DRIED	14.8	284	9.25	0.73	70.1
2	CINNAMON,GROUND	10.58	247	3.99	1.24	53.1
3	WHEAT, DURUM	9.89	216	15.55	4.25	42.8
4	OREGANO,DRIED	9.93	265	9	4.28	42.5
5	FENNEL SEED	8.81	345	15.8	14.87	39.8
6	CARAWAY SEED	9.87	333	19.77	14.59	38
7	BASIL, DRIED	10.35	233	22.98	4.07	37.7
8	CHIA SEEDS,DRIED	6.3	490	15.6	30.8	37.7
9	THYME,DRIED	7.79	276	9.11	7.43	37
10	PAPRIKA	11.24	282	14.14	12.89	34.9
11	CHILI POWDER	10.75	282	13.46	14.28	34.8
12	CLOVES,GROUND	9.87	274	5.97	13	33.9
13	Cocoa Powder	2.7	220	18.1	13.1	29.8
14	SPEARMINT,DRIED	11.3	285	19.93	6.03	29.8
15	PEPPERS,HUNGARIAN,RAW	14.84	345	12.35	15.85	26.8
16	PARSLEY,DRIED	5.89	292	26.63	5.48	26.7
17	PEPPER,BLACK	12.46	251	10.39	3.26	25.3
18	FENUGREEK SEED	8.84	323	23	6.41	24.6
19	RYE	10.75	325	15.91	2.22	23.8
20	SHALLOTS,RAW	4	341	8.1	1.49	23.6
21	PEPPERS,SERRANO,RAW	22.63	281	11.86	8.2	21.6
22	DILL SEED	7.7	305	15.98	14.54	21.1
23	TURMERIC,GROUND	11.36	354	7.83	9.88	21.1
24	RICE, WHITE,STMD,CHINESE RESTAURANT	6.13	316	13.35	20.85	21
25	POPPY SEED	5.95	525	17.99	41.56	19.5
26	NUTS, PISTACHIO NUTS,DRY RSTD,W/SALT	4.5	446	18.55	19.4	18.4
27	BUCKWHEAT FLR,WHOLE-GROAT	9	342	12.29	1.33	18.3
28	CAROB FLOUR	11.53	364	19.3	6.04	17.4
29	ARROWROOT FLOUR	9.44	354	12.48	2.3	17.3
30	PEANUT BUTTER,SMOOTH STYLE,W/ SALT	7.8	327	52.2	0.55	15.8
31	RADISHES,WHITE ICICLE,RAW	2	348	12.3	0.5	15.7
32	BARLEY,HULLED	10.09	352	9.91	1.16	15.6
33	MILLET,COOKED	6.55	246	17.3	7.03	15.4
34	OAT BRAN,RAW	6.5	246	17.3	7	15.4
35	ONION POWDER	5.39	341	10.41	1.04	15.2
36	RICE FLOUR,WHITE	10.6	338	10.34	1.63	15.1
37	TRITICALE	10.01	338	13.18	1.81	14.6
38	GINGER,GROUND	9.94	335	8.98	4.24	14.1
39	ROSEMARY,FRESH	67.77	131	3.31	5.86	14.1
40	PALM HEARTS,RAW	3.1	344	10.9	2.1	14
41	SESAME SEEDS,WHOLE,DRIED	3.3	565	16.96	48	14
42	THYME,FRSH	65.11	101	5.56	1.68	14
43	LOTUS SEEDS,RAW	1.7	594	18.17	49.9	13.7
44	WHEAT BRAN,CRUDE	11.12	360	23.15	9.72	13.2
45	SORGHUM FLR	12.42	332	9.61	1.95	13.1
46	BEANS, NAVY,MATURE SEEDS,CND	10.06	343	20.96	1.13	12.7
47	WHEAT,HARD WHITE	10.42	340	10.69	1.99	12.7
48	WHEAT,HARD RED WINTER	12.17	331	10.35	1.56	12.5
49	TOMATILLOS,RAW	14.56	258	14.11	2.97	12.3
50	MUSTARD SD,GROUND	5.27	508	26.08	36.24	12.2

TOP 100 FIBER-CONTAINING FOODS (51 - 100)

USDA Nutrition Database

	Shrt Desc	% Water	KCAL per 100 gm	% Protein As Is	% Fat As Is	% D. Fiber As Is
51	TRITICALE FLR,WHOLE-GRAIN	12.76	329	15.4	1.92	12.2
52	WHEAT,HARD RED SPRING	13.1	327	12.61	1.54	12.2
53	WHEAT,SOFT RED WINTER	9.57	342	11.31	1.71	12.2
54	RYE FLOUR,DARK	10.97	349	10.88	1.52	11.8
55	CHESTNUTS,EUROPEAN,RAW,PEELED	9.45	374	6.39	4.45	11.7
56	SUNFLOWER SD KRNLS,DRIED	1.2	582	19.33	49.8	11.1
57	BEANS, FAVA,IN POD,RAW	73.32	93	5.6	2.12	11
58	NUTS, HAZELNUTS OR FILBERTS	5.79	629	13.7	61.15	11
59	RICE FLOUR,BROWN	10	357	7.46	2.08	11
60	TOFU,SALTED&FERMENTED (FUYU)	8.43	347	24.33	1.31	11
61	SOYMILK,ORIGINAL & VANILLA,W/ ADDED CA,VITAMINS A & D	11.79	345	24.95	2.17	10.8
62	KAMUT,CKD	11.02	338	14.57	2.43	10.7
63	NUTS, PINE NUTS,DRIED	5.9	629	11.57	60.98	10.7
64	WHEAT GERM,CRUDE	10.74	340	13.21	2.5	10.7
65	EPAZOTE,RAW	70.78	103	4.71	2.75	10.6
66	ORANGE PEEL,RAW	72.5	97	1.5	0.2	10.6
67	BEANS, NAVY,MATURE SEEDS,RAW	63.81	140	8.23	0.62	10.5
68	NUTS, ALMONDS,DRY RSTD,W/SALT	2.8	607	21.23	55.17	10.5
69	BEANS, SML WHITE,MATURE SEEDS,RAW	63.24	142	8.97	0.64	10.4
70	BEANS, YEL,MATURE SEEDS,RAW	62.98	144	9.16	1.08	10.4
71	BUCKWHEAT	8.41	346	11.73	2.71	10.3
72	WHEAT FLOURS,BREAD,UNENR	12.11	345	10.5	1.6	10.1
73	BARLEY,PEARLED,COOKED	9.75	343	13.25	3.4	10
74	BEANS, CRANBERRY (ROMAN),MATURE SEEDS,RAW	64.65	136	9.34	0.46	10
75	BUCKWHEAT GROATS,RSTD,CKD	11.15	335	12.62	3.1	10
76	GRAPE LEAVES,RAW	76.1	69	4.27	1.97	9.9
77	NUTS, ALMONDS	4.51	590	21.4	52.52	9.9
78	NUTS, PISTACHIO NUTS,RAW	1.85	567	20.95	44.82	9.9
79	COCONUT H2O (LIQ FROM COCONUTS)	5.31	628	14.95	60.75	9.7
80	TEMPEH	5.16	486	34.54	20.65	9.6
81	PEANUTS,ALL TYPES,DRY-ROASTED,W/SALT	6.39	570	26.15	49.6	9.5
82	PECANS,DRY RSTD,W/SALT	1.13	715	9.2	75.23	9.5
83	BEANS, FRENCH,MATURE SEEDS,RAW	66.57	129	7.05	0.76	9.4
84	PEANUTS,ALL TYPES,CKD,BLD,W/SALT	1.45	599	28.03	52.5	9.4
85	PECANS	1.12	710	9.5	74.27	9.4
86	BEANS, KIDNEY,CALIFORNIA RED,MATURE SEEDS,RAW	66.93	124	9.13	0.09	9.3
87	BEANS, KIDNEY,ROYAL RED,MATURE SEEDS,RAW	66.99	123	9.49	0.17	9.3
88	QUINOA,CKD	10.95	337	14.7	2.2	9.1
89	BEANS, PINTO,MATURE SEEDS,RAW	62.95	143	9.01	0.65	9
90	COCONUT MEAT,RAW	47	354	3.3	33.5	9
91	GARLIC POWDER	6.45	331	16.55	0.73	9
92	NUTS, MACADAMIA NUTS,DRY RSTD,W/SALT	1.75	594	17.3	51.45	9
93	PEANUTS,SPANISH,RAW	1.78	579	28.01	49.04	8.9
94	PEANUTS,ALL TYPES,RAW	41.78	318	13.5	22.01	8.8
95	BEANS,BLACK, boiled without salt	65.74	132	8.86	0.54	8.7
96	NUTS, HICKORYNUTS,DRIED	1.36	718	7.91	75.77	8.6
97	CORN, HOMINY,CANNED,WHITE	8.67	378	11.02	4.22	8.5
98	CORN,WHITE	10.83	364	8.75	5.09	8.4
99	BEANS, BLACK TURTLE,MATURE SEEDS,RAW	65.74	130	8.18	0.35	8.3
100	PEAS,SPLIT,MATURE SEEDS,RAW	69.49	118	8.34	0.39	8.3

APPENDIX 3

Hi Fiber Chocolate Chip Cookies - Reduced Sugar			
The Biome Bakery TM			
	Percent	Grams	English
Whole Wheat flour	28.0	174	1 3/8 cups
Whole Eggs	8.7	54	1 Large Egg
Butter, Saltetd	18.0	112	1 stick
Baking Soda	0.54	3	1/2 teaspoon
Molasses	1.30	8	1 tablespoon
Polydextrose	16.0	99	3/4 cup
Vanilla ext	0.5	3	1/2 teaspoon
Choc Chips, 85%	27.0	167	1 cup
Total	100.0	620	

Procedure:
sift and dry blend flour with baking soda
Cream butter with polydextrose
add vanilla, molasses and egg to butter/polydextrose
Add flour/baking soda, and mix until smooth
Add Chips and mix gently to incorporate
Use a spoon or icecream scoop, to place 2 ounce dollops (60 grams) of batter onto parchment paper
bake 12 minutes on paper at 375 F Convection
makes 12, 50 gram cookies

This cookie makes it possible and healthy to snack. For me, being able to have an espresso and a cookie after dinner is part of making a diet sustainable.

The ingredients in this cookie contain only traces of sugar, except for the chocolate chips. Even an eighty-five percent cocoa chocolate contains about fifteen percent sugar, I only know one place to buy them online and they are expensive! The sixty percent cocoa chocolate contains almost forty percent sugar. These cookies, made with the eighty five percent cocoa chips contain about 5 grams of sugar per 50-gram cookie. And since the formula has about 14 grams of fat per 50-gram cookie, the rate of absorption of glucose into the bloodstream will be moderate, so you shouldn't see a big glucose spike after eating one of these. If you used the more popular semi-sweet chocolate chips, which are sixty percent cocoa, the sugar would go up to 6.5 grams per cookie. Not so bad. The best way to avoid the sugar is to substitute sunflower seeds for the chocolate chips. Quantity matters, when it comes to calories and blood glucose, so one cookie is good, two is pushing it and more is a problem!

If you want to reduce the sugar further, reduce or take out the chocolate chips. A good option is to replace the chocolate chips with sunflower seeds. They have great texture, flavor, fiber and fat.

Nutritional Profile – Chocolate Chip Cookie

	Weight (grams)	Calories	Protein (grams)	Total Fat (grams)	Saturated Fat (grams)	Omega-3 (grams)	Cholesterol (mg)	Total Carbs (grams)	Sugar (grams)	Fiber (grams)	Sodium (mg)	ORAC (umol TE)
Totals	50	210	2.9	14	8	0	40	25	4.5	10	135	5,500

APPENDIX 4

Oat Bran Cereal
April 25, 2017
L. Heflich

This is a good breakfast recipe, but it can be eaten anytime to get more fiber and antioxidants into your diet. It will raise your blood glucose due to the high carb content, but you can moderate this by adding some fat. Butter works great and tastes good, but I also use flax oil or coconut oil.

Ingredients:

40 grams (3 Tablespoons)	Oat bran cereal
13 grams (1 Tablespoon)	Chia seeds
7.4 grams (1 Tablespoon)	Cocoa powder
6 grams (1 Teaspoon)	Cinnamon powder
1 gram (1/3 Teaspoon)	Ginger powder
0.25 grams (1 Pinch)	Clove powder
45 ml (3 Tablespoons)	Milk or Half and Half (optional - it really helps the texture)
15 grams (1 Tablespoon)	Butter
225 ml (1 Cup)	Water

Procedure:

Sift cocoa powder, cinnamon powder, ginger powder, clove powder to remove lumps.

Mix all dry ingredients together in a cereal bowl.

You can use preheated hot water or cold water and microwave

Add half the water, stir with a spoon until smooth.

Add remaining water and stir until smooth.

If you used cold water, microwave on high for 2 minutes, stir and microwave for another minute.

Add oil or butter, and optional half and half and stir.

Let it sit a few minutes and eat.

Nutritional Profile – Oat Bran Cereal

	Weight (grams)	Calories	Protein (grams)	Total Fat (grams)	Saturated Fat (grams)	Omega-3 (grams)	Cholesterol (mg)	Total Carbs (grams)	Sugar (grams)	Fiber (grams)	Sodium (mg)	ORAC (umol TE)
Totals	300	305	11	20	9	1.9	32	39	1	13	135	13,890

If you want to eliminate the cholesterol, use coconut oil instead of butter. The added fat helps to moderate the absorption of glucose into the bloodstream, reducing the impact of the carbs in this meal on blood glucose.

APPENDIX 5

Kale and Eggplant Lasagna
April 25, 2017
L. Heflich

This is an easy and delicious way to get more fiber and antioxidants into your diet. I usually make a large baking dish of this recipe, and then after it cools, I cut it up into meal-sized pieces, refrigerate a couple to eat in the next few days and freeze the rest. It's a simple matter to reheat them in the microwave or oven when I need them.

Ingredients:

8 grams (2 cloves)	Garlic
300 grams (1 large)	white onion, diced
45 grams (4 tablespoons)	olive oil
250 grams (1 medium)	eggplant, cubed ½ inch
45 grams (3 tablespoons)	sundried tomatoes in oil, drained
15 grams (2 tablespoons)	turmeric powder
3 grams (1 teaspoons)	ginger powder
800 gms (3 cups)	tomato sauce
200 gms (1 bag! or 5 cups)	baby kale (can be frozen)

60 grams (6 tablespoons)	chia seeds
60 grams (6 tablespoons)	parmesan cheese, grated
200 gms (7 ounces)	cheese, sliced (mozzarella, Swiss, etc. all work well)
50 grams (5 tablespoons)	wheat germ

Eggplant Filling:

- Sauté in a covered pot with olive oil, minced garlic, diced onion and cubed eggplant until tender
- Add sundried tomatoes, turmeric and ginger and cook for another 10 minutes
- Mash together to form a uniform paste (put it into a food processor to make a really smooth paste)

Layering the Ingredients:

- Spread half of the tomato sauce on the bottom of a large 10 X 15 inch glass baking dish
- Sprinkle half of the chia seeds evenly on top of the tomato sauce
- Place a layer of half of the kale leaves, breaking up the leaves into pieces no bigger than 2 inches, removing any thick stems (this is especially easy if the kale is frozen)
- Evenly spread the eggplant filling over the kale, smoothing it with a spoon
- Spread the remaining tomato sauce on top of the eggplant filling layer
- Sprinkle the remaining chia seeds evenly on top of the tomato sauce
- Add another layer of the remaining kale leaves in the same manner as before
- Place a layer of sliced cheese on top of the kale

- Sprinkle evenly the grated parmesan cheese on top
- Last, sprinkle the wheat germ evenly on top to keep the cheese on top from burning in the oven

Bake:

Preheat oven to 350 Deg F
Bake for 1 hour

Serve:

Cut it up into squares, about 5 by 5 inches and place in bowls or covered containers. Serve immediately or refrigerate what you will eat within 48 hours, and freeze the rest.

Nutritional Profile – Kale Lasagna

	Weight (grams)	Calories	Protein (grams)	Total Fat (grams)	Saturated Fat (grams)	Omega-3 (grams)	Cholesterol (mg)	Total Carbs (grams)	Sugar (grams)	Fiber (grams)	Sodium (mg)	ORAC (umol TE)
Totals	339	384	17.5	23	17.5	1.8	35	31	4	10	225	7515

APPENDIX 6

Morning Kickstart

I call this recipe my Kickstart, because I take this in the morning on days when I am extending my fast until lunch. When I am fasting until lunch, the Kickstart helps me avoid eating. The Kickstart is high in fiber but is very low in sugar, which is what I want to avoid during my morning fast.

It contains fiber to feed the bacteria in the intestines, charcoal to absorb toxins in food to protect the good bacteria, and antioxidants to reduce inflammation. The oils will give you your daily requirement for linoleic and linolenic fatty acids, needed for a healthy gut. The L-Glutamine and psyllium feed and aid in developing the layer of bacteria in the intestinal wall. The Charcoal powder absorbs toxins in the food to prevent damage to the good bacteria. Cinnamon and Cocoa powder are high in dietary fiber and are also powerful antioxidants. Note that while beta glucan is one of the best dietary fibers for feeding beneficial bacteria, you shouldn't take more than a quarter gram per serving. That is too small to measure without an expensive analytical scale, but for 10 servings that's 2.5 grams or a teaspoon full.

You can make it by the serving, but I like to blend the dry ingredients in advance, enough to make 10 servings and mix it really well in a small container. Be careful to keep the lid tightly closed as it is dusty. It stores unrefrigerated and will keep for months. This way, when it's time to make the shake, I just spoon out what I need and don't have to measure all the ingredients each time.

Morning Kickstart Shake!

For One Serving	For 10 Servings	Ingredient
1 tablespoon	10 tablespoons	Psyllium husk fiber whole flake
1/2 teaspoon	5 tablespoons	cocoa powder
1 tablespoon	10 tablespoons	L-Glutamine (optional)
1/3 teaspoon	3 tablespoons	Charcoal powder (optional)
1/3 teaspoon	3 tablespoons	Cinnamon powder (optional)
1/10 teaspoon	1 teaspoon	beta glucan fiber (optional)

When you are ready to make the shake, take a glass of water (12 ounces), add two tablespoons of sour cream or unsweetened yogurt to improve the flavor and consistency. Stir in the dry ingredients. If you made the 10-serving mix, then you will need to add up what you put into it and divide by ten to get a single serving amount. You can use a blender or just mix it with a spoon. Then, while blending or stirring it, I dribble in a tablespoon of grapeseed oil and a teaspoon of flax seed oil. Drink this every morning and your intestines will send you a message – hopefully a happy one!

When I need to lose a few pounds, or compensate for a few meals where I let myself go, I will fast until lunch time and then take the Kickstart for my lunch. This way I can go until dinner time without taking in any substantial calories and no carbs. It's a great way to get back on track after a little binge, as the fiber and antioxidants are high, and the sugar and calories are very low.

REFERENCES

1   Jim Strole and Bernadeane, *Living Without Death: The Experience of Physical Immortality*, (Scottsdale, AZ: People Unlimited Inc., 1999)

2   Dr. Abdul Wahab Pathath, "Theories of Aging", *The International Journal of Indian Psychology*, Vol. 4(3), April-June, 2017, pages 15-22

3   Ernest Becker, *The Denial of Death*, (New York: The Free Press, 1973)

4   Mary Ann Bakerji, Milay Luis Lam, and Rochelle Chaiken, "Insulin Resistance and the Metabolic Syndrome", Chapter 37, in Leonid Poretsky, *Principles of Diabetes Mellitus, Third Edition*, (Cham, Switzerland: Springer International Publishing AG, 2017)

5   Collins, Jim and Porras, Jerry I, *Built to Last: Successful Habits of Visionary Companies,* (New York: HarperCollins Publishers, October 26, 1994)

6   Eckhart Tolle, *The Power of Now: A Guide to Spiritual Enlightenment*, (Novato, California: New World Library, 1997)

7   Dr. Stuart Brown, *Play: How It Shapes the Brain, Opens the Imagination, and Invigorates the Soul*, (New York: The Penguin Group, 2010)

8   Leonard W. Heflich, *Balanced Leadership: A Pragmatic Guide for Leading*, (Bloomington, Indiana: iUniverse Publishers, June, 2018)

9   Rachel Brazil, "Nocebo: the placebo effect's evil twin", *The Pharmaceutical Journal*, March 15, 2018, pages 1-11

10   Launa Colloca, "Nocebo effects can make you feel pain", *Science*, Vol 358, Issue 6359, October 6, 2017, Page 44

11   Bob Monroe Associates, Hemi-Sync by Monroe Products, Lovingston, VA 22949, www.hemi-sync.com

12   Dr. Thomas Cowan, *Human Heart, Cosmic Heart*, (White River Junction, Vermont: Chelsea Green Publishing, 2016)

13   "How Elements are Formed", *The Science Learning Hub*, www.sciencelearn.org.nz

14   Carlo Rovelli, *The Order of Time*, (New York: Riverhead Books, 2017)

15 Otto Siegel, Ph.D., personal communication, www.geniuscoaching.com

16 Tim Ferriss, *Tools of Titans: The Tactics, Routines, and Habits of Billionaires, Icons, and World-Class Performers*, (Boston: Houghton Mifflin Harcourt, December 6, 2016)

17 Valerie Ann Worwood, *The Complete Book of Essential Oils and Aromatherapy*, (Novato, California: New World Library, 2016)

18 Robert M. Pirsig, *Zen and the Art of Motorcycle Maintenance: An Inquiry into Values*, (New York: William Morrow and Company, 1974)

19 Astrid Kolderup and Birger Svihus, "Fructose Metabolism and Relation to Atherosclerosis, Type 2 Diabetes, and Obesity", *Journal of Nutrition and Metabolism*, Vol 2015, Article ID 823081, June 7, 2015

20 Peter J. Havel, DVM, PhD, "Dietary Fructose: Implications for Dysregulation of Energy Homeostasis and Lipid/Carbohydrate Metabolism", *Nutrition Reviews*, Vol. 63(5), May 2005, pages 133-157

21 Hope Jahren, *Lab Girl*, (New York: Alfred A. Knopf, 2016)

22 Scott M. Grundy, "Overnutrition, ectopic lipid and the metabolic syndrome", *J of Investig Medicine*, Vol. 64, 2016, pages 1082-1086

23 D. El Khoury, C. Cuda, B.L. Luhjovyy, and G.H. Anderson, "Beta Glucan: Health Benefits in Obesity and Metabolic Syndrome, A Review", *Journal of Nutrition and Metabolism*, Vo. 2012, Article ID 851362, 2012, pages 1-28

24 JM Keenan, JJ Pins, C Frazel, A Moran, and L Turnquist, "Oat ingestion reduces systolic and diastolic blood pressure in patients with mild or borderline hypertension: a pilot trial", *The Journal of Family Practice*, Vol 51(4), April 1, 2002, page 369

25 D. Gentilcore, R. Chaikomin, KL Jones, A. Russo, C. Feinle-Bisset, JM Wishart, CK Rayner, and M. Horowitz, "Effects of fat on gastric emptying of and the glycemic, insulin, and incretin responses to a carbohydrate meal in type 2 diabetes", *The Journal of Clinical Endocrinology and Metabolism*, Vol. 91, 2006, pages 2062-7

26 Felipe De Vadder, Petia Kovatcheva-Datchary, Daisy Goncalves, Jennifer Vinera, Carine Zitoun, Adeline Duchampt, Frederik Bäckhed and Gilles Mithieux, "Microbiota-Generated Metabolites Promote Metabolic Benefits via Gut-Brain Neural Circuits", *Cell*, Vol 156, January 16, 2014, pages 84-96

27 Manu S. Goyal, Siddarth Venkatesh, Jeffrey Milbrandt, Jeffrey I. Gordon, and Marcus E. Raichle, "Feeding the brain and nurturing the mind: Linking nutrition and the gut microbiota to brain development", *PNAS*, Vol 112(46), Oct. 6, 2015, pages 14105-14112

28 Megan W. Bourassa, Ishraq Alim, Scott J. Bultman and Rajiv R. Rutan, "Butyrate, neuroepigenetics and the gut microbiome: Can a high fiber diet improve brain health?", *Neuroscience Letters*, Vol. 625, 2016, pages 56-63

29 T.S. Dharmarajan, "Psyllium versus Guar Gum: Facts and Comparisons", *Practical Gastroenterology*, February 2005, pages 72-76

30 Steven R. Gundry, MD, *The Plant Paradox: The Hidden Dangers in "Healthy" Foods That Cause Disease and Weight Gain*, (New York: HarperCollins Publishers, 2017)

31 Mahesh S. Desai, Anna M. Seekatz, Nicole M. Koropatkin, Nobuhiko Kamada, Christina A. Hickey, Mathis Wolter, Nicholas A. Pudlo, Sho Kitamoto, Nicholas Terrapon, Arnaud Muller, Vincent B. Young, Bernard Henrissat, Paul Wilmes, Thaddeus S. Stappenbeck, Gabriel Nuñez, and Eric C. Martens, "A Dietary Fiber-Deprived Gut Microbiota Degrades the Colonic Mucous Barrier and Enhances Pathogen Susceptibility", *Cell*: 167, 2016, pages 1339-1353

32 Dr. Natasha Campbell McBride MD, MMedSci(neurology), MMedSci(nutrition), *Gut and Psychology Syndrome: Natural Treatment for Autism, Dyspraxia, A.D.D., Dyslexia, Depression, Schizophrenia*, (Cambridge, UK: Medinform Publishing, January 2017)

33 Mohamed Al-Saleh Ali, Barbera Corkey, Jude Deeney, Keith Tornheim and Ethan Bauer, "Effect of artificial sweeteners on insulin secretion, ROS, and oxygen consumption in pancreatic beta cells", *FASEB Journal*, Vol. 25, April 2011

34 Bianca Martins Gregório, Diogo Benchimol De Souza, Fernanda Amorim de Morais Nascimento, Leonardo Matta, and Caroline Fernandes-Santos, "The Potential Role of Antioxidants in Metabolic Syndrome", *Current Pharmaceutical Design*, Vol. 22(7), February 2016, pages 859-869

35 Sam Kean, *Caesar's Last Breath: Decoding the Secrets of the Air Around Us*, (New York: Little, Brown and Company, July 2017)

36 N Halberg, M Henriksen, N Söderhamm, B Stallknecht, T Ploug, P Schjerling and F Dela, "Effect of intermittent fasting and refeeding on insulin action in healthy men", *Journal of Applied Physiology*, Vol. 99(6), December, 2005, pages 2128-2136

37 LK Heilbronn, SR Smith, CK Martin, SD Anton and E. Ravussin, "Alternate-day fasting in nonobese subjects: effects on body weight, body composition, and energy metabolism", *American Journal of Clinical Nutrition*, Vol. 81(1), January, 2005, pages 69-71

38 Michael L. Dansinger, Joi Augustin Gleason, John L. Griffith, Harry P. Selker, and Ernst J. Shaefer, "Comparison of the Atkins, Ornish, Weight Watchers, and Zone Diets for Weight Loss and Heart Disease Risk Reduction", *Journal of the American Medical Association*, Vol. 293, No. 1, January 5, 2005, Pages 43-53

39 Dean Ornish, MD, "Was Dr. Atkins Right?", *Journal of the American Dietetic Association*, Vol 104(4), April 2004, 2004, pages 537-542

40 Dr. Michael Gershon, *The Second Brain: A Groundbreaking New Understanding of Nervous Disorders of the Stomach and Intestine*, (New York: HarperCollins Publishers Inc., November 17, 1999)

41 Mazen Alsahli, Muhammad Z. Shrayyef and John E. Gerich, "Normal Glucose Homeostasis", Chapter 2, in Leonid Poretsky, *Principles of Diabetes Mellitus, Third Edition*, (Cham, Switzerland: Springer International Publishing AG, 2017)

42 Romain Bouziathttp, Reinhard Hinterleitner, Judy J. Brown, Jennifer E. Stencel-Baerenwald, Mine Ikizler, Toufic Mayassi, Marlies Meisel, Sangman M. Kim, Valentina Discepolo, Andrea J. Pruijssers, Jordan D. Ernest, Jason A. Iskarpatyoti, Léa M. M. Costes, Ian Lawrence, Brad A. Palanski, Mukund Varma, Matthew A. Zurenski, Solomiia Khomandiak, Nicole McAllister, Pavithra Aravamudhan, Karl W. Boehme, Fengling Hu, Janneke N. Samsom, Hans-Christian Reinecker, Sonia S. Kupfer, Stefano Guandalini, Carol E. Semrad, Valérie Abadie, Chaitan Khosla, Luis B. Barreiro, Ramnik J. Xavier, Aylwin Ng, Terence S. Dermody, Bana Jabri; "Reovirus infection triggers inflammatory responses to dietary antigens and development of celiac disease"; *Science*, Volume 356, Issue 6333, April 7, 2017, pg. 44-50

43 Paddy C. Dempsey, Neville Owen, Thomas E. Yates, Bronwyn A. Kingwell, and David W. Dunstan, "Sitting Less and Moving More: Improved Glycaemic Control for Type 2 Diabetes Prevention and Management", *Current Diabetes Reports*, Vol. 16, October 3, 2016, page 114

44 Al Sears, M.D., *P.A.C.E.: The 12-Minute Fitness Revolution*, (Royal Palm Beach, FL: Wellness Research and Consulting, 2010)

45 Jeffrey F. Life, M.D., Ph.D., *The Life Plan: How Any Man Can Achieve Lasting Health, Great Sex, and a Stronger, Leaner Body*, (New York: Atria Books, 2011)

46 Christopher McDougall, *Born to Run: A Hidden Tribe, Superathletes, and the Greatest Race the World Has Never Seen*, (New York: Alfred A. Knopf, 2009)

47 GBD 2015 Disease and Injury Incidence and Prevalence, Collaborators, "Global, regional, and national incidence, prevalence, and years lived with disability for 310 diseases and injuries, 1990-2015: a systematic analysis for the Global Burden of Disease Study 2015", *Lancet (London, England).* **388** (10053), October 8, 2016, pages 1545-1602.

48 Marcia F. Kalin, Marcus Goncalves, Jennifer John-Kalarickal, and Vivian Fonseca, "Pathogenesis of Type 2 Diabetes Mellitus", Chapter 15, in Leonid Poretsky, *Principles of Diabetes Mellitus, Third Edition,* (Cham, Switzerland: Springer International Publishing AG, 2017)

49 Rebekah Gospin, James P. Leu, and Joel Zonszein, "Diagnostic Criteria and Classification of Diabetes", Chapter 8, in Leonid Poretsky, *Principles of Diabetes Mellitus, Third Edition,* (Cham, Switzerland: Springer International Publishing AG, 2017)

50 Jim. I. Mann and Alexandra Chisholm, "Dietary management of diabetes mellitus in Europe and North America", *International Textbook of Diabetes Mellitus, Fourth Edition,* Page 577 – 588, Edited by Ralph A. DeFronzo, Ele Ferrannini, Paul Zimmet and K. GeorgeM. M. Alberti, (Chichester, UK: John Wiley and Sons, Ltd., 2015)

51 George F. Inglett, United States Patent Number 4,996,063, February 26, 1991

52 Richard D. Feinman, Ph.D., Wendy K. Pogozelski Ph.D., Arne Astrup M.D., Richard K. Bernstein M.D., Eugene J. Fine M.S., M.D., Eric C. Westman M.D., M.H.S., Anthony Accurso M.D., Lynda Frassetto M.D., Barbara A. Gower Ph.D., Samy I. McFarlane M.D., Jörgen Vesti Nielsen M.D., Thure Krarup M.D., Laura Saslow Ph.D., Karl S. Roth M.D., Mary C. Vernon M.D., Jeff S. Volek R.D., Ph.D., Gilbert B. Wilshire M.D., Annika Dahlqvist M.D., Ralf Sundberg M.D., Ph.D., Ann Childers M.D., Katherine Morrison M.R.C.G.P., Anssi H. Manninen M.H.S., Hussain M. Dashti M.D, Ph.D., F.A.C.S., F.I.C.S., Richard J. Wood Ph.D., Jay Wortman M.D., Nicolai Worm Ph.D., "Dietary carbohydrate restriction as the first approach in diabetes management: Critical review and evidence base", *Nutrition* Vol. 31, 2015, pages 1-13

53 Megan L. Gow, Sarah P. Garnett, Louise A. Baur, Natalie B. Lister, "The Effectiveness of Different Diet Strategies to Reduce Type 2 Diabetes Risk in Youth", *Nutrients, Vol.* 8(8), 2016, page 486

54 S.H. Knudsen, L.S. Hansen, M. Pedersen, T. Dejgaard, J. Hansen, and G.V. Hall, "Changes in insulin sensitivity precede changes in body composition during 14 days of step reduction combined with overfeeding in healthy young men", *J. Applied Physiology,* Vol. 113, 1985, pages 7-15

55   Amalia Gastaldelli, "Insulin resistance and reduced metabolic flexibility: cause or consequence of NAFLD?", *Clinical Science*, Vol. 131, 2017, pages 2701-2705

56   P. Würsch, FX Pi-Sunyer, "The role of viscous soluble fiber in the metabolic control of diabetes. A review with special emphasis on cereals rich in beta-glucan", *Diabetes Care*, Vol 20(11), Nov. 1, 1997, pages 1774-1780

57   Nadine E. Palermo and Michael F. Holick, "Role of Vitamin D in the Pathogenesis of Diabetes", Chapter 7, in Leonid Poretsky, *Principles of Diabetes Mellitus, Third Edition*, (Cham, Switzerland: Springer International Publishing AG, 2017)

58   A.C. Martin, R.A. Sanders, and J.B. Watkins III, "Diabetes, Oxidative Stress and Antioxidants: A Review", *J. Biochem Molecular Toxicology*, Vol. 17, Number 1, 2003, pages 24-38

59   Keith Richards, with James Fox, *Life*, (New York, Little, Brown and Company, 2010)

60   Patience Gray, *Honey From a Weed*, (London: Prospect Books, March 3, 2001)

61   James Strole and Bernadeane, with Joe Bardin, *Just Getting Started: Fifty years of living FOREVER, Insights on agelessness and immortality*, (Phoenix, AZ: Author2Market Division of D&L Press, July 2017)

62   David Foster Wallace, *Infinite Jest*, (New York: Little, Brown and Company, 1996)

63   Llyn Roberts and Robert Levy, *Shamanic Reiki: Expanded Ways of Working with Universal Life Force Energy*, (Winchester, UK: O-Books, 2008)